PERFORMING PREVENTIVE SERVICES

A Bright Futures Handbook

EDITORS

Susanne Tanski, MD, MPH, FAAP

Lynn C. Garfunkel, MD, FAAP

Paula M. Duncan, MD, FAAP

Michael Weitzman, MD, FAAP

FUNDED BY

The Commonwealth Fund

PUBLISHED BY

American Academy of Pediatrics
DEDICATED TO THE HEALTH OF ALL CHILDREN™

American Academy of Pediatrics Department of Marketing and Publications

Maureen DeRosa, MPA, Director, Department of Marketing and Publications

Mark Grimes, Director, Division of Product Development

Amy Pirretti, MS, Staff Editor, Department of Community and Specialty Pediatrics

Sandi King, MS, Director, Division of Publishing and Production Services

Maryjo Reynolds, Product Manager, Bright Futures

Kate Larson, Manager, Editorial Services

Kevin Tuley, Director, Division of Marketing and sales

Performing Preventive Services: A Bright Futures Handbook
Library of Congress Control Number: 2008922528
ISBN: 978-1-58110-522-3
BF0036

The recommendations in this publication do not indicate an exlusive course of treatment or serve as a standard of medical care. Variations, taking into account individual circumstances, may be appropriate.

Brand names are furnished for identification purposes only. No endorsement of the manufacturers or products mentioned is implied.

Every effort has been made to ensure that the drug selection and dosage set forth in this text are in accordance with the current recommendations and practice at the time of publication. It is the responsibility of the health care provider to check the package insert of each drug for any change in indications and dosage and for added warnings and precautions.

Please note: The American Academy of Pediatrics is not responsible for the content of the resources mentioned in this publication. Inclusion in this publication does not imply an endorsement by the American Academy of Pediatrics. Web site addresses are as current as possible, but may change at any time.

CONTENTS

CONTRIBUTORS

Joel L. Bass, MD, FAAP
Pediatrician, Pediatric Ambulatory Care Center
Newton-Wellesley Hospital
Newton, MA
Bicycle Helmets

Dana Best, MD, MPH, FAAP
Director, The Smoke Free Project
Children's National Medical Center
Associate Professor of Pediatrics
George Washington University School of Medicine
    and Health Sciences
Washington, DC
Tobacco Smoke Exposure and Tobacco Use Cessation

Suzanne C. Boulter, MD, FAAP
Pediatrician, NH Dartmouth Family Medical Program
Concord Hospital Family Health Center
Concord, NH
Fluoride Varnish Application Tips

Robert S. Byrd, MD, MPH
Associate Professor of Clinical Pediatrics
UC Davis Medical Center
Sacramento, CA
Parental Health Literacy

Stephen Cook, MD, MPH, FAAP
Assistant Professor of Pediatrics
University of Rochester School of Medicine and Dentistry
Rochester, NY
Cardiometabolic Risk of Obesity

Terry C. Davis, PhD
Professor of Medicine and Pediatrics
Louisiana State University Health Sciences Center
Shreveport, LA
Parental Health Literacy

Monte A. DelMonte, MD, FAAP
Pediatric Ophthalmology & Adult Strabismus
    Kellogg Eye Center
Skillman Professor of Pediatric Ophthalmology
Professor, Ophthalmology and Visual Sciences
Professor, Pediatrics and Communicable Diseases
    University of Michigan
Ann Arbor, MI
Vision

Joseph DiFranza, MD
Professor of Family Medicine and Community Health
University of Massachusetts Medical School
Worcester, MA
Tobacco Dependence

Benard P. Dreyer, MD, FAAP
Professor of Pediatrics
NYU School of Medicine
New York, NY
Child and Adolescent Depression

Paula Duncan, MD, FAAP
Youth Health Director, Vermont Child Health
    Improvement Program
Clinical Professor of Adolescent Medicine, Department
    of Pediatrics
University of Vermont College of Medicine
Burlington, VT
Developmental Strengths

Burton Edelstein, DDS, MPH
Pediatric Dentist, Professor of Dentistry
Director, Division of Community Health
    Columbia University School of Dental and Oral
    Surgery
    New York, NY
Founding Director, Board Chair
    Children's Dental Health Project
    Washington, DC
Early Childhood Caries

Ann Clock Eddins, PhD, MBA, CCC-A
Departments of Audiology and Otolaryngology
University of Rochester Medical Center
Rochester, NY
Hearing

Joy Gabrielli, MA
Research Assistant, CeASAR
Children's Hospital Boston
Boston, MA
Adolescent Alcohol and Substance Use and Abuse

Lynn C. Garfunkel, MD, FAAP
Pediatrician
　　Rochester General Pediatric Associates
Associate Professor of Pediatrics, Associate Program
　　Director,
Pediatric and Combined Medicine-Pediatric Training
　　Programs
University of Rochester School of Medicine
Rochester, NY
Assessing Growth and Nutrition
*Immunizations, Newborn Screening, and Capillary
　　Blood Tests*

Frances Page Glascoe, MD
Division of Child Development, Department of Pediatrics
Vanderbilt University School of Medicine
Nashville, TN
Developmental and Behavioral Considerations

Sandra G. Hassink, MD, FAAP
Director, Nemours Obesity Intiative
A I DuPont Hospital for Children
Wilmington, DE
Weight Maintenance and Weight Loss

Amy M. Heneghan, MD, FAAP
Pediatrician, Palo Alto Medical Foundation
　　Palo Alto, CA
Adjunct Associate Professor of Pediatrics
Case Western Reserve University
Rainbow Babies and Children's Hospital
　　Cleveland, OH
Maternal Depression

Marcia E. Herman-Giddens, PA, DrPH
Child and Family Health Consultant
Adjunct Professor, School of Public Health,
　　UNC Chapel Hill
President, Tick-borne Infections Council of
　　North Carolina, Inc
Sexual Maturity Stages

Paul B. Kaplowitz, MD, FAAP
Chief of Endocrinology, Children's National Medical Center
Professor of Pediatrics
　　George Washington University School of Medicine
　　and Health Sciences
Washington, DC
Sexual Maturity Stages

Alex Kemper, MD, MPH, MS, FAAP
Department of Pediatrics/Community and Family
　　Medicine
Duke Clinical Research Institute
Duke University
Durham, NC
Vision

John R. Knight, MD
Associate Professor of Pediatrics, Harvard Medical School
Director, CeASAR, Children's Hospital Boston
Boston, MA
Adolescent Alcohol and Substance Use and Abuse

Marc Lande, MD
Associate Professor of Pediatrics
University of Rochester School of Medicine and Dentistry
Rochester, NY
Blood Pressure

Amy Pirretti, MS
Manager, Bright Futures Materials Development
Department of Community and Specialty Pediatrics
American Academy of Pediatrics
Elk Grove Village, IL
Developmental Strengths

Donna Phillips, MD
Assistant Professor of Orthopedic Surgery
NYU Langone Medical Center
New York, NY
Intoeing and Outtoeing

Mary Lou Popolizio, MS, PNP
Pediatric Nurse Practitioner, "Don't Weight" Program
　　Coordinator
Rochester General Pediatric Associates
　　Rochester General Hospital
Adjunct Faculty
　　University of Rochester School of Nursing
Rochester, NY
Weight Maintenance and Weight Loss

Timothy Roberts, MD, MPH, FAAP
Pediatrician, Adolescent Medicine
Brooke Army Medical Center
Fort Sam Houston, TX
Adolescent Alcohol and Substance Use and Abuse

Edward L. Schor, MD, FAAP
Vice President
The Commonwealth Fund
New York, NY
Priorities in Well-Child Care

Robert P. Schwartz, MD
Professor of Pediatrics, Chief of Pediatric Endocrinology
Wake Forest University School of Medicine
Winston Salem, NC
Motivational Interviewing

Eric Small, MD, FAAP
Clinical Assistant Professor of Pediatrics, Orthopedics,
    and Rehabilitation Medicine
Mt. Sinai School of Medicine
New York, NY
Sports Participation

Victor C. Strasburger, MD, FAAP
Chief of the Division of Adolescent Medicine
Professor of Pediatrics, Professor of Family & Community
    Medicine
University Of New Mexico
Albuquerque, NM
Children, Adolescents, and Media

Susanne Tanski, MD, MPH, FAAP
Pediatrician, Children's Hospital
    Dartmouth-Hitchcock Medical Center
    Lebanon, NH
Assistant Professor of Pediatrics
    Dartmouth Medical School
    Hanover, NH
Assessing Growth and Nutrition
Immunizations, Newborn Screening, and Capillary
    Blood Tests

Danielle Thomas-Taylor, MD, MPH, FAAP
Clinical Senior Instructor, Department of Pediatrics
    University of Rochester Medical Center
Pediatrician, Rochester General Pediatric Associates
    Rochester General Hospital
Rochester, NY
Intimate Partner Violence

Shari Van Hook, PA-C, MPH
Director of Research Operations
Center for Adolescent Substance Abuse Research
Children's Hospital Boston
Adolescent Alcohol and Substance Use and Abuse

William Varade, MD
Associate Professor
Department of Pediatrics, Nephrology
University of Rochester School of Medicine and Dentistry
Rochester, NY
Blood Pressure

Stuart Weinstein, MD, FAAP
Pediatric Orthopaedic Surgery and Spinal Deformity
Ignacio V. Ponseti Chair and Professor of Orthopaedic
    Surgery
Department of Orthopedics and Rehabilitation
University of Iowa Hospitals and Clinics
Iowa City, IA
Spine, Hip, and Knee

Michael Weitzman, MD, FAAP
Professor of Pediatrics and Psychiatry
New York University School of Medicine
New York, NY
Foreword

Robert Wellman, PhD, CAS
Professor of Behavioral Sciences
    Fitchburg State College
    Fitchburg, MA
Adjunct Professor of Family Medicine and Community
    Health
    University of Massachusetts Medical School
    Worcester, MA
Tobacco Dependence

Mark Wolraich, MD, FAAP
Professor of Behavioral Pediatrics
University of Oklahoma College of Medicine
Oklahoma City, OK
Disruptive Behavior Disorders

Susan M. Yussman, MD, MPH, FAAP
Assistant Professor of Pediatrics and Community Health
Division of Adolescent Medicine
University of Rochester School of Medicine and Dentistry
Rochester, NY
Cervical Dysplasia
Sexually Transmitted Infections

FOREWORD

This book is addressed and dedicated to those health professionals who provide our children with their preventive health care services. It has been designed to accompany the newly revised Bright Futures Guidelines published by the American Academy of Pediatrics. In fact, those individuals who wrote and edited the new Bright Futures Guidelines spent countless hours offering the editors of this book useful guidance and reviewing multiple drafts, and for this we are truly grateful. This book has been designed to provide guidance about how best to actually provide the preventive services suggested in the Bright Futures Guidelines. Nationally renowned experts were chosen to review the scientific and medical literature about the most effective and efficient ways to deliver the preventive services suggested by the Bright Futures Guidelines.

The content of this book has been arranged for ease of use and to accompany the Bright Futures Guidelines. Topics vary from how to perform and bill for office-based screening for vision and hearing, obesity and its complications, child development, depression, and behavior problems, to tobacco dependence and parental literacy or depression, as well as how to provide counseling about topics critical to children's health and development. It has been designed for ease of use as well as to offer the very best suggestions about how to provide our children with the very best preventive services currently available. If it helps those clinicians providing these vitally important services, we will have achieved what we set out to do. Good luck!

Michael Weitzman, MD, Editor

EDWARD L. SCHOR, MD

PRIORITIES IN WELL-CHILD CARE

Well-child care accounts for 25% of visits to primary care practitioners for children younger than 15 and 40% for children younger than 1 year.[1] These visits constitute a large percentage of pediatricians' time, with the average time for preventive care visits ranging from 16 to 19 minutes[2–4] (slightly more for adolescent visits[5]).

Although pediatricians and parents are generally satisfied with the time available for these visits,[4] some ambivalence remains. Most pediatricians (53%) report that they have enough time,[6] but many say lack of time (85%) and the need to prioritize among preventive care topics (47%) are barriers to implementing recommended preventive care services.[5] Parents do not always have sufficient time to have their needs fully addressed. Though most (88%) report having enough time during preventive care visits, a significant number of parents (34%) say they were not able to ask all of their questions.[7]

Responding to the Population Served

Pediatricians individualize care by making choices about what to include and omit during well-child care visits. Little information is available about what guides these decisions but, ideally, pediatricians are considering (1) the needs of the families and community they serve, (2) the needs of the child and family, (3) the outcomes they intend to achieve, and (4) the preferences of the parents and child.

Successful pediatric practices prioritize care based on a general understanding of their patient populations. This means they are able to respond not only to the needs of individual families, but also to the community as a whole. Practices can structure their care to be efficient and effective by knowing the demographics of the families they serve, the resources available in their community, and through relationships with other professionals who serve or care for their patients.

Meeting the specific needs of the individual child and family requires that the practitioner first gather information and then provide services that are appropriate for the child's level of risk and development. Some information is obtained through standardized assessments, with a special focus on child development and behavior and the psychosocial issues faced by the family. In general, lower-risk families receive services primarily intended to promote optimal development to prevent the onset of illness or injury. Higher-risk families may receive similar primary prevention services and, in addition, are given detection and intervention services to reduce the likelihood of health or developmental problems becoming clinically apparent. Preventive care for children with established, chronic problems should also include services to minimize the progression of their conditions so they do not further limit the child's physical, emotional, or social functioning.[8]

Making the Most of the Well-Child Care Visit

Decisions regarding which issues to address must be made jointly by the family and the health care practitioner. Research has shown that patient satisfaction and compliance increase when the patient—or the patient and family—play an active role in determining the purpose of the visit, identifying problems of concern, and planning a management strategy.[9] Given the many services available during a well-child visit, patients and parents can help prioritize by identifying topics that need not be covered.

To further prioritize among the possible care options in a time-limited visit, the family and health care practitioner should agree on the specific, desired outcomes of the visit and of well-child care during the current developmental stage. In general, the outcomes of well-child care include

- The child's physical health and development

- Emotional, social, and cognitive development

- The family's capacity and functioning

Although outcomes can focus on both the long and short term, it is important to remember that well-child care can affect the seemingly distant future for both child and family. For example, altering dietary habits in childhood or adolescence can help prevent heart attacks during middle age. Positive parenting can avoid adult depression and substance abuse.[10] Researchers are increasingly recognizing the importance and impact of early life experience and health behaviors on health and well-being in later life.[11]

Alternatively, short-term outcomes focus on current development. In early childhood, one outcome of well-child care is being ready for school entry. According to a recent consensus document, school readiness includes the 6 domains of physical well-being; social, emotional, cognitive, and language development; and acquisition of general knowledge.[12]

Building on these concepts, Box 1 proposes outcomes of well-child care that should be achieved by or for children by the time they are 5 years old. Not all of these outcomes are the sole responsibility of the pediatric practitioner.

The outcomes in italics are ones to which *well-child care ideally should contribute, but for which it should not be held accountable.* During well-child care visits, the practitioner should determine how the child and family are progressing toward the desired outcomes. Specifying the outcomes for well-child care, assessing progress, and using the outcomes to help prioritize the content of care will help improve the quality and value of preventive pediatric care. It is the equivalent of developing a care management plan for children with acute or chronic health problems.

What About Evidence?

Some argue that one way to prioritize the content of well-child care is to only offer services that have evidence of effectiveness. Although this approach may be effective in other areas of pediatric care, much of well-child care has not been subjected to the scrutiny of researchers.[13] Further, most of the existing research does not adhere to high methodological standards.[14] Some important preventive services have been studied, however, and found effective, and should be provided in accordance with the recommendations cited in Box 1.[15,16] Even when evidence supports the provision of a service, individual differences in patients' or parents' receptivity and in the practitioners' skills may limit its effectiveness.

Changing the Structure of Well-Child Care

Providing appropriate and effective well-child care efficiently will require systemic changes in how that care is organized.[17] Some suggestions include

- Improve appointment and reminder systems to reduce missed appointments and wasted time. Mail and telephone reminders can improve appointment-keeping. Advanced access systems decrease the interval between when appointments are made and when they occur.

- Waiting time should be reduced and used in a structured way to collect clinical data. The time patients spend alone in waiting rooms and examination rooms is approximately equal to the time they spend with clinical staff.[18]

Box 1. Outcomes of Well-Child Care at Age 5

Physical Health and Development

- No undetected hearing problem
- No undetected vision problem/normal vision or corrected optimally
- No chronic health problem without a management plan (eg, asthma, neuromotor disability)
- Immunization complete for age
- No undetected lead poisoning
- No undetected congenital anomalies/birth defects
- *No untreated dental caries*
- *Good nutritional habits and no obesity; attained appropriate growth and weight*
- *No exposure to tobacco smoke*
- *Physically safe environments for living and traveling*

Emotional, Social, and Cognitive Development

- No unrecognized or untreated developmental delays (ie, emotional, social, cognitive, communication)
- *Child has good self-esteem*
- *Child recognizes relationship between letters and sounds*
- *Child has positive social behaviors with peers and adults*

Family's Capacity and Functioning

- Parents are knowledgeable about child's physical health status and needs
- No unrecognized maternal depression, family violence, or family substance use
- No undetected early warning signs of child abuse or neglect
- Parents feel valued and supported as child's primary caregiver and function in partnership with the child's health care practitioner
- Parents understand and are able to fully use well-child care services
- *Parents read regularly to the child*
- *Parents are knowledgeable and skilled to anticipate and meet a child's developmental needs*
- *Parents have access to consistent sources of emotional support*
- *Parents are linked to all appropriate community services*

- A variety of screening instruments is available to assess biopsychosocial risks and strengths, health and developmental status, and health behaviors. These instruments should be used routinely, according to a schedule appropriate to the age and circumstances of the patients and their families. Some of this information is available during the prenatal period and should be obtained then, if possible.

- Health records should be computerized, but even hard copy records should include preventive services summary sheets to prompt clinical staff to provide essential services and record their provision.

- The schedule for well-child care should be individualized, and the contents of preventive care packaged into a series of modules. The provision of these modules will be determined by the patient's age, health status, previously received services, biopsychosocial risks, and the desired outcomes of care as determined jointly by the health care practitioner and family.

- At the conclusion of a well-child care visit, the family should receive an explicit care plan, including any necessary referrals and follow-up.

- Practices must know the referral resources in their community and have an organized approach to using them.

- Finally, responsibility for the various processes involved in well-child care should be reviewed by each practice and assigned to the staff member best able to complete that task effectively and efficiently.

References

1. Hing E, Cherry DK, Woodwell DA. National ambulatory medical care survey: 2003 summary. *Adv Data.* 2005;(365):23–24

2. LeBaron CW, Rodewald L, Humiston S. How much time is spent on well-child care and vaccinations? *Arch Pediatr Adolesc Med.* 1999;153:1154–1159

3. Norkin Goldstein EN, Dworkin PH, Bernstein B. Time devoted to anticipatory guidance during child health supervision visits: how are we doing? *Ambul Child Health.* 1999;5:113–120

4. Olson LM, Inkelas M, Halfon N, Schuster MA, O'Connor KG, Mistry R. Overview of the content of health supervision for young children: reports from parents and pediatricians. *Pediatrics.* 2004;113:1907–1916

5. American Academy of Pediatrics Division of Health Policy Research. Periodic Survey of Fellows: Executive Summary. Periodic Survey #56. Pediatricians' Provision of Preventive Care and Use of Health Supervision Guidelines. American Academy of Pediatrics Web Site. 2004. http://www.aap.org/research/periodicsurvey/ps56exs.htm

6. Cheng TL, DeWitt TG, Savageau JA, O'Connor KG. Determinants of counseling in primary care pediatric practice: physician attitudes about time, money, and health issues. *Arch Pediatr Adolesc Med.* 1999;153:629–635

7. Halfon N, Inkelas M, Mistry R, Olson LM. Satisfaction with health care for young children. *Pediatrics.* 2004;113:1965–1972

8. E. Schor. Should Children with Special Health Care Needs Have Separate Preventive Care Visits? *Arch Pediatr Adolesc Med.*

9. Starfield B, Steinwachs D, Morris I, Bause G, Siebert S, Westin C. Patient-doctor agreement about problems needing follow-up visit. *JAMA.* 1979;242:344–346

10. Felitti VJ, Anda RF, Nordenberg D, et al. Relationship of childhood abuse and household dysfunction to many of the leading causes of death in adults: the Adverse Childhood Experiences (ACE) study. *Am J Prev Med.* 1998;14(4):245–258

11. Halfon N, Hochstein M. Life course health development: an integrated framework for developing health, policy, and research. *Milbank Q.* 2002;80(3):433–479

12. Rhode Island KIDS COUNT. *Getting Ready: Findings from the National School Readiness Indicators Initiative: A 17-State Partnership.* Providence, RI: Rhode Island KIDS COUNT; 2005

13. R. D. Sege and E. De Vos, Evidence-Based Health Care for Children: What Are We Missing?, The Commonwealth Fund, April 2010.

14. Moyer VA, Butler M. Gaps in the evidence for well-child care: a challenge to our profession. *Pediatrics.* 2004;114(6):1511–1521

15. Regalado M, Halfon N. Primary care services promoting optimal child development from birth to age 3 years. *Arch Pediatr Adolesc Med.* 2001;155:1311–1322

16. Gielen AC, McDonald EM, Wilson MEH, et al. Effects of improved access to safety counseling, products, and home visits on parents' safety practices: results of a randomized trial. *Arch Pediatr Adolesc Med.* 2002;156:33–40

17. D. Bergman, P. Plsek, and M. Saunders, A High-Performing System for Well-Child Care: A Vision for the Future, The Commonwealth Fund, October 2006

18. American Academy of Pediatrics Division of Health Policy Research. Periodic Survey of Fellows: Executive Summary. Periodic Survey #43—Part 1. Characteristics of Pediatricians and Their Practices: The Socioeconomic Survey. American Academy of Pediatrics Web Site. 2000. http://www.aap.org/research/periodicsurvey/ps43aexs.htm

HISTORY, OBSERVATION, AND SURVEILLANCE

Each Bright Futures visit begins with 3 interrelated components—history, observation, and surveillance. History sets the stage for the visit. It allows health care professionals to assess strengths, accomplish surveillance, and enhance understanding of the child and family. Observation allows the professional to assess interactions between parent and child. Surveillance permits the professional to track the acquisition of developmental milestones and strengths over time.

The chapters in this section of the book focus on topics that often emerge during this portion of the visit. Several, such as **Intimate Partner Violence** and **Parental Health Literacy,** deal with sensitive topics for which health care professionals might find additional guidance useful. Others, such as **Maternal Depression, Disruptive Behavior Disorders, Child and Adolescent Depression,** and **Tobacco Dependence,** explore issues that must be spotted early so as to enhance the likelihood of successful intervention. **Developmental Strengths** focuses on the strengths and skills that lay the foundation for a healthy adulthood.

BENARD DREYER, MD

CHILD AND ADOLESCENT DEPRESSION

What Is Childhood and Adolescent Depression?

Common Signs and Symptoms in Infants and Preschoolers

- Apathy
- Withdrawal from caregivers
- Delay or regression in developmental milestones
- Failure to thrive without organic cause
- Excessive crying
- Dysregulation
- Irritability

Common Signs and Symptoms in School-Aged Children[1]

- Low self-esteem
- Excessive guilt
- Somatic complaints, such as headaches and stomachaches
- Anxiety, such as school phobia or excessive separation anxiety
- Irritability
- Sadness
- Isolation
- Anger
- Bullying
- Fighting

- Fluctuating moods
- Sleep disturbance
- Academic decline

Common Signs and Symptoms in Adolescents

Signs and symptoms of depression in adolescents are similar to those in adults and, according to the *Diagnostic and Statistical Manual, Fourth Edition, Text Revision (DSM-IV-TR),*[2] include

- Depressed or irritable mood
- Loss of interest or pleasure in activities
- Feelings of worthlessness or excessive guilt
- Low energy/fatigue; psychomotor retardation
- Insomnia or hypersomnia; appetite and weight changes
- Poor concentration
- Thoughts of death or suicide

Causes of adolescent depression are complex. Although genetic factors are important, the onset of a depressive episode may be precipitated by difficult or stressful life experiences, such as family, school, or peer relationship problems. Sexual or physical abuse also is a risk factor.[3]

Why Is It Important to Include Childhood and Adolescent Depression in History, Observation, and Surveillance?

Major depression in children and adolescents is a relatively common disorder. Major depressive disorder is estimated to occur in 1% of preschoolers and 2% of school-aged children. Evidence also indicates that the prevalence is increasing, with onset at earlier ages.[3] Studies also show that 4% to 6% of adolescents may experience depression at any one time, with lifetime prevalence rates by late adolescence of 20% to 25%.[3]

Depression in prepubertal children occurs equally in males and females.[3] Adolescents are different, with depressive disorders after puberty occurring in twice as many females as males.[3]

Depression is related to serious morbidity and mortality.[4] Depressed children and adolescents frequently have comorbid mental disorders, such as

● Anxiety disorders

● Attention-deficit/hyperactivity disorder

● Disruptive disorders, including conduct disorder and oppositional defiant disorder (see the "Disruptive Behavior Disorders" chapter for more information on these disorders)

● Eating disorders[2]

Depressed adolescents are at higher risk of alcohol and substance abuse. Generally depression precedes the onset of alcohol and substance abuse by 4 to 5 years, so identification of depression may provide an opportunity for prevention.[1] Depressed adolescents also experience significant impairment in school functioning and in interpersonal relationships.

Adolescents who are depressed also are at increased risk of suicide ideation, suicide attempts, and completed suicides. Studies show that 85% of depressed teenagers report suicidal ideation and 32% attempt suicide. Approximately 60% of adolescents who commit suicide have a depressive disorder.[3] Depression in prepubertal children has a lower rate of suicide (0.8 per 100,000).[3]

Suicide is the third leading cause of death in youth aged 15 to 19. More than 1,600 youth (aged 15 to 19) committed suicide in 2000.[5] Suicide is the fourth leading cause of death in youth aged 10 to 14. In this age group, 5 times as many males as females completed a suicide attempt.

Depression among adolescents is likely to continue and may lead to other mental disorders. Studies indicate that 20% to 40% of adolescents with a major depressive episode go on to develop bipolar disorder within 5 years.[1]

Moreover, depression in adolescents is likely to continue into adulthood. Approximately 70% will have another episode of depression in 5 years. Teenagers with depression are 4 times as likely as others to have depression as adults.[3]

Depression is underdiagnosed. Studies show that only 50% of adolescents with depression are diagnosed.[6]

Should You Screen for Depression?

In 2007 the American Academy of Pediatrics endorsed the Guidelines for Adolescent Depression in Primary Care, which recommend primary clinicians assess for depression in adolescents at high risk and those presenting with emotional problems.

The US Preventive Services Task Force (USPSTF), in 2009, recommended screening "adolescents (12–18 years of age) for major depressive disorder when systems are in place to ensure accurate diagnosis, psychotherapy (cognitive-behavioral or interpersonal), and follow-up." There was insufficient evidence for the USPSTF to recommend screening children (aged 7–11).

In 2010 the American Academy of Pediatrics released a supplement to *Pediatrics, Enhancing Pediatric Mental Health Care: Report from the American Academy of Pediatrics Task Force on Mental Health* and *Addressing Mental Health Concerns in Primary Care: A Clinician's Toolkit,* which provides pediatric health care practitioners guidance on how to select appropriate assessment, screening, and surveillance instruments (available at: http://pediatrics.aappublications.org/conten/vol125/supplement_3).

A number of depression screening tools for children and adolescents have been evaluated. Some of the more widely used assessments and tools are highlighted below.

Beck Depression Inventory (BDI), Beck Depression Inventory for Primary Care (BDI-PC), Center for Epidemiological Studies–Depression Scale (CES-D), and Center for Epidemiological Studies–Depression Scale for Children (CES-DC)[7]

The Agency for Healthcare Research and Quality[8] conducted a systematic evidence review of these depression screening tools in children and adolescents.

The review indicated that

- These tools perform reasonably well in community adolescent populations.

- They have sensitivities that range from 75% to 100% and specificities from 49% to 90%.

- The positive predictive values of these tests are low due to the lower specificity and the low prevalence of depression in these populations (most of the patients identified are not depressed[8]).

- The CES-D, while not validated for children younger than 12 years, has been used in several studies involving children as young as 10 years.

Similar evidence regarding operating characteristics of depression screening tools is available in a recent review by Sharp and Lipsky.[9]

The Patient Health Questionnaire for Adolescents (PHQ-A) and the Patient Health Questionnaire (PHQ-9) Quick Depression Assessment

These screening tools

- Have sensitivities of 73% and specificities of 94% to 98% for the diagnosis of major depressive disorder in adolescents

- Have not been validated in preadolescent children

- Have positive predictive values of 40% to 60% depending on the prevalence of depression in the adolescent population being screened (this is due to the higher specificity of these screening tests, at the expense of a somewhat lower sensitivity)

An advantage of the PHQ-A is that it also assesses dysthymic disorder and other common mental health problems of adolescents. The advantage of the PHQ-9 is that it is very short (9 questions).[10,11]

Children's Depression Inventory (CDI),[12] Child Depression Scale (CDS), Children's Self-Report Rating Scale (CSRS), Depression Self-Rating Scale (DSRS), and Reynolds Adolescent Depression Scale (RADS)

These screening tools for depression in children and adolescents have been tested only in referred populations, and their use in primary care populations as general screening tools is untested.[8]

Pediatric Symptom Checklist and the Child Behavior Checklist (CBCL)

These general behavioral symptom checklists are good for highlighting psychosocial issues but are not appropriate for identifying the specific diagnosis of depression.[13]

How Should You Perform a Depression Screening?

Although screening for depression in preadolescent children is not specifically recommended in Bright Futures, a behavioral and psychosocial assessment is recommended at every visit. Some specific signs and symptoms of depression in children may be different from those in adolescents, but some overlap exists and you may wish to ask many of the same questions noted here for adolescents.

Perform a Preliminary Assessment Using HEADSS

At every health supervision visit with an adolescent, take a thorough psychosocial history based on the HEADSS method of interviewing. This method has recently been expanded to HEEADSSS (or HE^{2}ADS^3).

This assessment includes questions related to the following HE^{2}ADS^3 psychosocial domains.[14–16] Sample question topics are listed. For a complete list, see Goldenring and Rosen.[14]

Home: Who lives with the teen? What are relationships like at home? Recent moves or running away?

Education/Employment: School/grade performance—any recent changes? Suspension, termination, dropping out?

Eating: Likes and dislikes about one's body? Any recent changes in your weight or appetite? Worries about weight?

Activities: With peers and family? Church, clubs, sports activities? History of arrests, acting out, crime?

Drugs: Use of tobacco, alcohol, or drugs by peers, by teen, by family members?

Sexuality: Orientation? Degree and types of sexual experience and acts? Number of partners? Sexually transmitted infections, contraception, pregnancy/abortion?

Suicide/Depression:

- Feeling sad

- Sleep disorders (insomnia or hypersomnia)

- Feelings of boredom, helplessness, or hopelessness

- Emotional outbursts and impulsive behavior

- Withdrawal/isolation from peers and family

- Psychosomatic symptoms

- Decreased affect on interview

- Preoccupation with death (music, art, media)

- Suicidal ideation

- History of past suicide attempt, depression, or psychological counseling

- History of depression, bipolar disorder, or suicide in family or peers

Safety: History of accidents, physical or sexual abuse, or bullying? Violence in home, school, or neighborhood? Access to firearms?

To help you with your HEADSS/HE²ADS³ assessment, you also may want to use the Guidelines for Adolescent Preventive Services (GAPS) self-report questionnaires. These instruments, developed by the American Medical Association, are available for younger and middle-older adolescents in both English and Spanish.[17,18] Have adolescents fill out the GAPS form before you talk with them.

Take Additional Steps if Needed

Consider an adolescent at high risk of depression if the HEADSS/HE²ADS³ interview reveals any of the following:

- Any positive answers in the suicide/depression domain

- Poor or absent relationships with peers or family members

- History of acting out or antisocial behavior

- Recent deterioration in school performance

- Changes in appetite/weight

- Alcohol or substance abuse

- Recurrent serious accidents

- History of sexual or physical abuse

- Comorbid disorders, such as ADHD, anxiety disorders, conduct disorder, or oppositional defiant disorder

If you determine that an adolescent is at high risk on the basis of HEADSS/HE²ADS³ interviews, GAPS questionnaires, or comorbid mental disorders, consider using a standardized screening tool to assess adolescent symptoms of depression.

What Should You Do With an Abnormal Result?

Interview all adolescents who have a positive screen for depression.

Assess them for depressive symptoms and functional impairment based on the *DSM-IV-TR* criteria for major depressive disorder, dysthymia, and depression not otherwise specified.

Assess for comorbid conditions, both medical and psychiatric.

Perform a safety assessment for suicide risk.

- Does the adolescent now have suicidal thoughts or plans?

- Have prior attempts occurred?

- Does the plan or previous attempt have significant lethality or efforts to avoid detection?

- Has the adolescent been exposed to suicide attempt/completion by peers or family members?

- Does the adolescent have alcohol or substance abuse problems?

- Does the adolescent have a conduct disorder or patterns of aggressive/impulsive behavior?

- Does the family show significant family psychopathology, violence, substance abuse, or disruption?

- Does the adolescent have the means available (especially firearms and toxic medications)?

Meet with the adolescent's family members or caregivers.

Discuss a referral to a mental health professional. Make an immediate referral to a mental health provider or emergency services if severe depression, psychotic, or suicidal ideation/risk is evident.[19]

Educate adolescents and their family about depression and treatment options.

- Stress that depression is treatable.

- Briefly discuss treatment options, such as watchful waiting for mild depression, psychotherapy (cognitive behavioral therapy or interpersonal therapy), and medication (selective serotonin reuptake inhibitors).

- Encourage families to remove firearms and toxic substances from the house, especially if any suicidal ideation is present.

Provide information about print or online resources that may be helpful to adolescents and their families.

Schedule a follow-up visit in 1 to 2 weeks.

What Results Should You Document?

Document HEADSS/HE[2]ADS[3] assessment, scores of depression screening tools, referrals discussed or made, and follow-up plans.

ICD-9-CM Codes	
296.2x–296.3x	Major depressive disorder
300.4	Dysthymic disorder
309.0	Adjustment disorder with depressed mood
311	Depressive disorder, not otherwise specified

The American Academy of Pediatrics publishes a complete line of coding publications, including an annual edition of *Coding for Pediatrics*. For more information on these excellent resources, visit the American Academy of Pediatrics Online Bookstore at **www.aap.org/bookstore/**.

Resources

Scales and Tools

A number of good standardized screening tools exist for adolescent depression.

Beck Depression Inventory-II (BDI-II)

- 21-question, self-report questionnaire

- Updated version of Beck Depression Inventory; based on *DSM-IV-TR* criteria

- Appropriate for middle-older adolescents

- Available in Spanish
  Must be purchased from http://www.musc.edu/dfm/RCMAR/Beck.html

Center for Epidemiological Studies Depression Scale (CES-D)

- 20-question, self-report questionnaire developed for adults

- Appropriate for middle-older adolescents

- Available in Spanish
  Available free from http://www.hepfi.org/nnac/pdf/sample_cesd.pdf

Center for Epidemiological Studies Depression Scale for Children (CES-DC)

- 20-question, self-report questionnaire similar to the CES-D

- Appropriate for younger adolescents

- Available free from http://www.brightfutures.org/mentalhealth/pdf/professionals/bridges/ces_dc.pdf

Patient Health Questionnaire Adolescent Version (PHQ-A)

- 83-question, self-report questionnaire that screens for major depressive disorder, dysthymia, minor depressive disorder, anxiety disorders, drug abuse or dependence, nicotine dependence, and eating disorders

- First 16 questions focus on depression and mood and could be used without rest of questionnaire

- Moderately complex scoring schema

Patient Health Questionnaire Quick Depression Screen (PHQ-9)

- 9-question, self-report questionnaire that screens for major depressive disorder and other depressive disorder

- Does not screen for dysthymia

- Easy to score

- Available in Spanish
  Available for review at http://www.mapi-trust.org/questionnaires/66

Other depression screening tools

- Children's Depression Inventory (CDI)

- Reynolds Adolescent Depression Scale (RADS)

Interview Tools

Guidelines for Adolescent Preventive Services (GAPS): http://www.ama-assn.org/ama/pub/physician-resources/public-health/promoting-healthy-lifestyles/adolescent-health/guidelines-adolescent-preventive-services.shtml

Books

Berman AL, Jobes DA, Silverman MM. *Adolescent Suicide: Assessment and Intervention*. 2nd ed. Washington, DC: American Psychological Association; 2005

Empfield M, Bakalar N. *Understanding Teenage Depression: A Guide to Diagnosis, Treatment, and Management*. New York, NY: Henry Holt and Company; 2001

Fassler DG, Dumas L. *Help Me, I'm Sad: Recognizing, Treating, and Preventing Childhood and Adolescent Depression*. New York, NY: Penguin Books; 1998

Goodyer IM, ed. *The Depressed Child and Adolescent*. New York, NY: Cambridge University Press; 2001

King RA, Apter A, eds. *Suicide in Children and Adolescents*. New York, NY: Cambridge University Press; 2003

Koplewicz H. *More Than Moody: Recognizing and Treating Adolescent Depression*. New York, NY: Perigree Trade; 2003

Morris TL, March JS, eds. *Anxiety Disorders in Children and Adolescents*. 2nd ed. New York, NY: The Guilford Press; 2004

Miller, JA. *The Childhood Depression Sourcebook*. Chicago, IL: McGraw-Hill Professional; 1999

Article

US Preventive Services Task Force. Screening and treatment for major depressive disorder in children and adolescents: US Preventive Services Task Force Recommendation Statement. *Pediatrics*. 2009;123(4): 1223–1228

Web Sites

American Academy of Child & Adolescent Psychiatry

The Anxious Child: http://www.aacap.org/galleries/FactsForFamilies/47_the_anxious_child.pdf

American Academy of Pediatrics: Depression and Suicide: http://www.aap.org/healthtopics/depression.cfm

Bright Futures in Practice: Mental Health

Common Signs of Depression in Children and Adolescents: http://www.brightfutures.org/mentalhealth/pdf/families/bridges/dep_signs.pdf

Symptoms of Depression in Children and Adolescents: http://www.brightfutures.org/mentalhealth/pdf/families/ad/dep_symptoms.pdf

TeensHealth: http://www.kidshealth.org/teen/your_mind/feeling_sad/depression.html

Maternal and Child Health Bureau: http://www.mchlibrary.info/KnowledgePaths/kp_Mental_Conditions.html.

Mayo Clinic: http://www.mayoclinic.com/invoke.cfm?id=AN00685

National Alliance on Mental Illness: www.nami.org

National Institute of Mental Health: www.nimh.nih.gov

Mental Health America: http://www.mentalhealthamerica.net

NYU Child Study Center: http://www.aboutourkids.org

References

1. Birmaher B, Ryan ND, Williamson DE, et al. Childhood and adolescent depression: a review of the past 10 years. Part I. *J Am Acad Child Adolesc Psychiatry*. 1996;35:1427–1439

2. American Psychiatric Association. *Diagnostic and Statistical Manual of Mental Disorders*. 4th ed. Text rev. Washington, DC: American Psychiatric Publishing, Inc; 2000

3. Hatcher-Kay C, King CA. Depression and suicide. *Pediatr Rev*. 2003;24:363–371

4. American Academy of Child and Adolescent Psychiatry. Practice parameters for the assessment and treatment of children and adolescents with depressive disorders. *J Am Acad Child Adolesc Psychiatry*. 1998;37:63S–83S

5. National Institute of Mental Health. *In Harms Way: Suicide in America*. Bethesda, MD: National Institute of Mental Health, National Institutes of Health, US Department of Health and Human Services; 2003. NIH Publication No. 03-45940

6. Kessler RC, Avenevoli S, Ries Merikangas K. Mood disorders in children and adolescents: an epidemiologic perspective. *Biol Psychiatry*. 2001;15:1002–1014

7. Fendrich M, Weissman MM, Warner V. Screening for depressive disorder in children and adolescents: validating the Center for Epidemiological Studies Depression Scale for Children. *Am J Epidemiol*. 1990;131:538–551

8. Pignone M, Gaynes BN, Rushton JL, et al. *Screening for Depression. Systematic Evidence Review No. 6*. Rockville, MD: Agency for Healthcare Research and Quality; 2002. AHRQ Publication. No. 02-S002

9. Sharp LK, Lipsky MS. Screening for depression across the lifespan: a review of measures for use in primary care settings. *Am Fam Physician*. 2002;66:1001–1008

10. Johnson JG, Harris ES, Spitzer RL, Williams JB. The Patient Health Questionnaire for Adolescents: validation of an instrument for the assessment of mental disorders among adolescent primary care patients. *J Adolesc Health*. 2002;30:196–204

11. Spitzer RL, Johnson JG. *The Patient Health Questionnaire. Adolescent Version*. Biometrics Research Unit: New York State Psychiatric Institute; 1995

12. Kovacs M. *Children's Depression Inventory Manual*. North Tonawanda, NY: Multi-Health Systems, Inc; 1992

13. Stancin T, Palermo TM. A review of behavioral screening practices in pediatric settings: do they pass the test? *J Dev Behav Pediatr*. 1997;18:183–194

14. Goldenring J, Rosen DS. Getting into adolescent heads: an essential update. *Contemp Pediatr*. 2004;21:64

15. Goldenring JM, Cohen E. Getting into adolescent heads. *Contemp Pediatr*. 1988;5:75

16. Cohen E, MacKenzie RG, Yates GL. HEADSS, a psychosocial risk assessment instrument: implications for designing effective intervention programs for runaway youth. *J Adolesc Health*. 1991;12:539–544

17. American Medical Association. *Guidelines for Adolescent Preventive Services (GAPS): Recommendations Monograph*. Chicago, IL: American Medical Association; 1997

18. Levenberg PB. Elster AB. *Guidelines for Adolescent Preventive Services (GAPS): Implementation and Resource Manual*. Chicago, IL: American Medical Association; 1995

19. American Academy of Pediatrics Committee on Adolescence. Suicide and suicide attempts in adolescents. *Pediatrics*. 2000;105;871–874

PAULA DUNCAN, MD
AMY PIRRETTI, MS

DEVELOPMENTAL STRENGTHS

While developmental surveillance is relatively clear for young children (assessment of motor, social, and language skills), the details of promoting healthy development for school-aged children and adolescents is less well defined. In the third edition of the Bright Futures Guidelines, the visit priorities address healthy development and the Association of Maternal and Child Health Programs framework was adopted as a guide. This Strengths Assessment and Promotion framework provides a platform to accentuate what is going right for a child, and has a positive focus to health promotion and disease prevention. In addition, the concept of using a strength-based approach with children, youth, and families was recommended in all editions of Bright Futures. This chapter gives some ideas about implementing that recommendation in the primary care setting.

Why Is It Important to Include Developmental Strengths in History, Observation, and Surveillance?

Across all socioeconomic and racial/ethnic groups, the presence of assets or strengths is positively linked with increased healthy behaviors and fewer risk behaviors.[1,2] Incorporating strengths assessment and promotion in the primary care office setting can facilitate discussion of positive changes, and offer parents a strategy for effective communication with their child.[3]

Incorporating strengths assessment and promotion adds an important dimension to risk prevention. Prevention efforts oriented solely toward stopping or preventing a particular unhealthy behavior are not universally effective.[4,5] Furthermore, simply because children refrain from risky behavior does not mean they are healthy or accomplishing essential developmental tasks. A child who is "problem-free" isn't necessarily fully prepared for adulthood.[6]

Along with messages about what to avoid, children and parents should receive acknowledgement of healthy steps already taken.

Strengths assessment and promotion has a diverse research base. Practitioner recommendations supporting positive development have been informed by the research on prevention, resiliency, identity development, social development, and self-determination.

Researchers and practitioners in psychology, sociology, and social work have identified personal, environmental, and social assets that enable healthy and successful transition from childhood, through adolescence, and into adulthood.[7]

The Search Institute identified 40 assets in 8 categories of strengths and, since 1997, has published extensive data on their role in supporting successful development.[8]

A 1997 analysis by Resnick et al[9] of the National Longitudinal Study on Adolescent Health found that parent-family connectedness and perceived school connectedness protect against every health risk behavior measured except history of pregnancy.

Since 1981, the University of Washington Social Development Research Group has engaged in a longitudinal study testing strategies for reducing childhood risk factors for school failure, drug abuse, and delinquency. Their data support the long-term, protective influence of 2 key protective factors: (1) bonding to prosocial family, school, and peers and (2) clear standards or norms for behavior.[10]

This approach has support from agencies and organizations. In 2002, for example, the US Department of Health and Human Services endorsed strengths promotion in the document *Toward a Blueprint for Youth: Making Positive Youth Development a National Priority.*[11] States and communities are implementing programs to encourage positive youth development.

In 2005 the Association of Maternal and Child Health Programs adopted positive youth development as one of the guiding principles for the development of policies and programs to maximize the health of adolescents.[12]

The National Research Council and Institute of Medicine Committee on Community-level Programs for Youth conducted a 2-year study of the literature and research on strengths promotion.[13] It endorsed a summary list of "key youth assets" and developed a "provisional list of features of daily settings that are important for adolescent development."[13]

How Can You Assess Progress on Developmental Tasks and Promote Strengths in School-Aged Children and Adolescents?

Assessing Progress

- For each visit for school-aged and adolescent youth there are 5 priorities for anticipatory guidance at each visit. (box in next column).

Assess Strengths

- Practitioners have found it easier to provide comprehensive risk and developmental strengths screening if they use a framework or prompt.

- Ask questions about and record what is going well for the patient. For example,

11- to 14-Year Visit Priorities for the Visit

The first priority is to address the concerns of the adolescent and his parents. In addition, the Bright Futures Adolescence Expert Panel has given priority to the following additional topics for discussion in the 4 Early Adolescence Visits. The goal of these discussions is to determine the health needs of the youth and family that should be addressed by the health care professional. The following priorities are consistent throughout adolescence. However, the questions used to effectively obtain information and the anticipatory guidance provided to the adolescent and family can vary.

Including all the priority issues in every visit may not be feasible, but the goal should be to address issues important to this age group over the course of the 4 visits. These issues include:

- Phyisical growth and development (physical and oral health, body image, healthy eating, physical activity)

- Social and academic competence (connectedness with family, peers, and community; interpersonal relationships; school performance)

- Emotional well-being (coping, mood regulation and mental health, sexuality)

- Risk reduction (tobacco, alcohol, or other drugs; pregnancy; STIs)

- Violence and injury prevention (safety belt and helmet use, substance abuse and riding in a vehicle, guns, interpersonal violence [fights], bullying)

Source: Hagan Jf, Shaw Js, Duncan Pm, eds. 2008. Bright Futures. Guidelines for Infants, Children, and Adolescents, Third Edition. Elk Grove Village, IL: American Academy of Pediatrics

▶ What's been going well for you?

▶ What have you been doing to stay healthy?

▶ What do you like about yourself?

▶ What are you good at?

▶ What do you do to help others?

▶ Who are the important adults in your life?

H	**H**ome belonging (connection) decision-making
E	**E**ducation mastery (competence)
E	**E**ating
A	**A**ctivities physical activity, helping others
D	**D**rugs
S	**S**exual Activity
S	**S**uicide (mental health) coping, resilience, self-confidence
S	**S**afety

Source: Reif, CJ, Elster, AB, Adolescent Preventive Services. *Primary Care: Clinics in Office Practice.* Vol 25, NO1. March 1998. WB Saunders, Philadelphia, PA Goldenring JM, Cohen E. Getting into adolescent heads. *Contemp Pediatr.* 1988;5(7):75–90.

▶ If I were an employer, what are all the things that would make me want to hire you?

The commonly used HEEADSSS (**H**ome environment, **E**ducation and employment, **E**ating, peer-related **A**ctivities, **D**rugs, **S**exuality, **S**uicide/depression, and **S**afety from injury and violence) assessment also can elicit information about things that are "going well," such as a supportive home environment or success in school. Adopting the HEADSSS assessment by adding the specific concepts of independent decision-making to the Home component; helping others to the Activities component; and coping, resilience, and self-confidence to the Suicide or mental health component makes it a match for the Bright Futures visit priorities and developmental surveillance recommendations.

While the HEEADSSS pneumonic is mostly used with adolescent encounters, this approach can be modified to be consistent with Bright Futures and used with school-aged children.

Healthy behavior choices that present as negative replies to certain risk screening questions may also indicate strengths. For example, not smoking or refraining from unsafe sexual activity can be signs of independence, peer support, and/or good decision-making skills.

Seek out what strengths are present, rather than only looking for what might be missing.

Several strength assessment frameworks have been developed to provide shorthand descriptions of what a strong, well-rounded youth or adolescent "looks" like. The frameworks synthesize research on the supports, personal qualities, and experiences necessary for healthy development, and tend to echo one another. Examples follow.

- The **Circle of Courage** model for resiliency emphasizes generosity, independence, mastery, and belonging (GIMB).[14] The "GIMB" acronym was adopted for use by pediatricians, family physicians, and nurse practitioners who participated in the Vermont Youth Health Improvement Initiative.

- The Search Institute's **40 Developmental Assets** fit into 8 categories: support, empowerment, expectation/boundaries, educational competence, values, social competencies, and positive identity.[9]

- **The 5 Cs** (contribution, confidence, competence, connection, and character) were developed by the Forum for Youth Investment.[15]

- Social development theorists Ryan and Deci[16] identify **competence, autonomy,** and **relatedness** as essential for positive social development and personal well-being.

In 2005 the Association of Maternal and Child Health Programs identified the developmental tasks of adolescence, which were subsequently adopted by the Bright Futures Guidelines.[12]

Surveillance of Developement

The developmental tasks of middle adolescence can be addressed through information obtained in the medical examination, by observation, by asking specific questions, and through general discussion. The following areas can be assessed to better understand the developmental health of the adolescent. A goal of this assessment is to determine the adolescent is developing in an appropriate fashion and, if not, to provide information for assistance or intervention. In the assessment, determine whether the adolescent is making progress on these developmental tasks.

- Demonstrates physical, cognitive, emotional, social, and moral competencies

- Engages in behaviors that promote wellness and contribute to a healthy lifestyle

- Forms a caring, supportive relationship with family, other adults, and peers

- Engages in a positive way in the life of the community

- Displays a sense of self-confidence, hopefulness, and well-being

- Demonstrates resiliency when confronted with life stressors

- Demonstrates increasingly responsible and independent decision-making[11]

The National Research Council/Institute of Medicine's list of "Features of Positive Developmental Settings," a chapter in the manual *Community Programs to Promote Youth Development* (see Resources section of this chapter), can guide efforts to develop a strength-based office setting. Practical implications of the list for the pediatric office include using age-appropriate decorations, offering age-appropriate reading materials, and posting community volunteer opportunities.

Promote Strengths

- Model, and encourage your office colleagues to model, a positive, affirming approach toward children and adolescents.

- Briefly talk with patients and families about their particular strengths or about strengths in general.

- Adopt a shared decision-making strategy to encourage positive change when needed.

What Should You Do With an Abnormal Result?

All patients have strengths as well as areas requiring further attention for development.

Congratulate the patient and parent on the strengths that are present.

Offer anticipatory guidance that promotes additional strengths/assets. Even if you do not use an assessment framework, you can provide general guidance and encouragement.

Be aware that families and individuals may differ in their opinions of what constitutes a display of positive development. For example, assertiveness usually is

regarded as a sign of competence in many families, but it may be interpreted as a problem behavior in other cultures. Be respectful and ready to accommodate different perspectives.

Use shared decision-making (eg, motivational interviewing) to identify steps the child or parent can take to make positive change. See the "Motivational Interviewing" chapter for more information.

What Results Should You Document?

Record findings in the patient's chart and note at each visit whether the patient is making progress on the developmental tasks.

Customize your office encounter forms, previsit interview forms, and other materials to document all screenings and responses, and to begin discussions with patients. An example of a **practitioner reminder sticker** illustrated below was used in a preventive services quality improvement project as a prompt and documentation tool.

Practitioner Reminder Sticker for Patient Charts

Date of Screening
_____

Check Indicates a Preventive Screening

- [ ] Nutrition/Physical Activity
- [ ] Substance Abuse
- [ ] Sexual Activity
- [ ] Violence/Injury Prevention
- [ ] Oral Health

Emotional Wellbeing/MH

- [ ] Coping/Resiliency
- [ ] Competence (School)
- [ ] Connectedness (Family, Peers, Community)
- [ ] Decision-making
- [ ] Self-confidence/Hopefulness
- [ ] Puberty/Sexuality

CRAFFT? [ ] Yes [ ] No   2+ or –

Office Intervention   **Referral**

Source: Adapted from VCHIP

Resources

Books

Benson PL, Galbraith J, Espeland P. *What Kids Need to Succeed: Proven, Practical Ways to Raise Good Kids.* Minneapolis, MN: Free Spirit Publishing; 1994

Ginsburg KR, Jablow M. *A Parent's Guide to Building Resilience in Children and Teens: Giving Your Child Roots and Wings.* Elk Grove Village, IL: American Academy of Pediatrics; 2006

National Research Council and Institute of Medicine. *Community Programs to Promote Youth Development.* Committee on Community-Level Programs for Youth. Eccles J, Gootman JA, eds. Board on Children, Youth, and Families, Division of Behavioral and Social Sciences and Education. Washington, DC: National Academy Press; 2002. http://books.nap.edu/openbook.php?record_id=10022&page=R1

Simpson AR. *Raising Teens: A Synthesis of Research and a Foundation for Action.* Boston, MA: Center for Health Communication, Harvard School of Public Health; 2001

Articles

Duncan PM, Garcia AC, Frankowski BL, et al. Inspiring healthy adolescent choices: a rationale for and guide to strength promotion in primary care. *J Adolesc Health.* 2007;41(6):525–535

Frankowski BL, Leader IC, Duncan PM. Strength-based interviewing. *Adolesc Med State Art Rev.* 2009;20(1):22–40, vii–viii

Ginsburg KR. Engaging adolescents and building on their strengths. *Adolescent Health Update.* 2007;19

Web Sites

Administration for Children and Families: http://www.acf.hhs.gov/

National Clearinghouse on Families and Youth: http://ncfy.acf.hhs.gov/

The Search Institute: www.search-institute.org

The Seattle Social Development Research Group: www.sdrg.org

References

1. Sesma A Jr, Roehlkepartain EC. Unique strengths, shared strengths: developmental assets among youth of color. *Search Inst Insights Evid.* 2003;1(2):1–13

2. Oman R, Vesely S, Aspy C, McLeroy K, Rodine S, Marshall L. The potential protective effect of youth assets on adolescent alcohol and drug use. *Am J Public Health.* 2004;94:1425–1430

3. Jewiss J. *Qualitative Evaluation of the Vermont Youth Health Initiative.* Burlington, VT: Vermont Child Health Improvement Project; 2004

4. Blum RW, McCray E. *Youth Health and Development: Conceptual Issues and Measurement.* Presented at: WHO Meeting on Adolescent Health and Development; February 1999; Washington, DC

5. Catalano RF, Berglund ML, Ryan JAM, Lonczak HS, Hawkins JD. *Positive Youth Development in the United States: Research Findings on Evaluations of Positive Youth Development Programs.* United States Department of Health and Human Services Web Site. 1998. www.aspe.hhs.gov/hsp/positiveyouthdev99. Accessed January 20, 2006

6. Pittman KJ. *Promoting Youth Development: Strengthening the Role of Youth-Serving and Community Organizations.* Report prepared for The US Department of Agriculture Extension Services. Washington, DC: Center for Youth Development and Policy Research; 1991

7. Small S, Memmo M. Contemporary models of youth development and problem prevention: toward an integration of terms, concepts, and models. *Fam Relat.* 2004;53:3–11

8. Benson PL, Leffert N, Scales PC, Blyth DA. Beyond the village rhetoric: creating healthy communities for children and adolescents. *Appl Dev Sci.* 1998;2:138–159

9. Resnick MD, Bearman PS, Blum RW, Bauman KE, et al. Protecting adolescents from harm. Findings from the National Longitudinal Study on Adolescent Health. *JAMA.* 1997;278:823–832

10. Pittman K, Irby M, Tolman J, Yohalem N, Ferber T. *Preventing Problems, Promoting Development, Encouraging Engagement: Competing Priorities or Inseparable Goals?* Washington, DC: The Forum for Youth Investment, Impact Strategies, Inc; 2003

11. US Department of Health and Human Services, Administration for Children and Families, Family and Youth Services Bureau. *Toward a Blueprint for Youth: Making Positive Youth Development a National Priority.* National Clearing House on Families and Youth Web Site. 2001. http://www.ncfy.com/publications/pdf/blueprint.pdf. Accessed January 20, 2006

12. Association of Maternal and Child Health Programs and the National Network of State Adolescent Health Coordinators. *A Conceptual Framework for Adolescent Health.* The Annie E. Casey Foundation Web Site. 2005. http://www.amchp.org/aboutamchp/publications/conc-framework.pdf. Accessed February 3, 2006

13. Eccles J, Gootman J, eds. Board of Children, Youth and Families, Division of Behavioral and Social Sciences, National Research Council, Institute of Medicine. *Community Programs To Promote Youth Development*. Washington, DC: The National Academy Press; 2002. www.nap.edu/books/0309072751/html. Accessed January 20, 2006

14. Catalano RF, Hawkins JD. The social development model: a theory of antisocial behavior. In: Hawkins JD, ed. *Delinquency and Crime: Current Theories*. New York, NY: Cambridge University Press; 1996:149–197

15. Brendtro L, Brokenleg M, Van Bockern S. *Reclaiming Youth At Risk: Our Hope for the Future*. Bloomington, IN: Solution Tree; 2002

16. Ryan RM, Deci EL. Self-determination theory and the facilitation of intrinsic motivation, social development, and well-being. *Am Psychol*. 2000;55:68–78

MARK WOLRAICH, MD

DISRUPTIVE BEHAVIOR DISORDERS

Bright Futures consistently emphasizes family-centered care, including the mental health of the entire family unit. As such, it is important to incorporate screening and surveillance for issues related to behavior and mental health into routine pediatric care. Primary care practitioners are often the first and only contact for families that are struggling with behavior or mental health problems, and there are insufficient numbers of child psychiatrists, child psychologists, and social workers. Further, social stigma and financial constraints (for families and practitioners) often prevent families seeking help from mental health professionals. Parents may think problems will get better by themselves or that they should be strong enough to handle them on their own, and thus may be unlikely to bring up the topic on their own.

What Are Disruptive Behavior Disorders?

A spectrum of diseases and disease severities exist within disruptive behavior disorders. Children with disruptive disorders can be inattentive, hyperactive, aggressive, and/or defiant. They may repeatedly defy societal rules of their own cultural group or disrupt the classroom or other environments.

Attention-Deficit/Hyperactivity Disorder (ADHD)

Attention-deficit/hyperactivity disorder is the most commonly diagnosed neurobehavioral disorder of childhood. Symptoms include hyperactivity, impulsivity, and inattention. Subtypes include combined type, primarily inattentive, and primarily hyperactive. Children with primarily inattentive type may miss early detection and may therefore incur greater dysfunction.

Boys are 4 times more likely to have ADHD than girls. Etiology is most likely multifactorial; neurotransmitter deficits, genetics, and perinatal complications have been implicated. Although environmental factors may contribute to the severity of problems, they are not considered etiologic by themselves.

Oppositional Defiant Disorder (ODD)

Oppositional defiant disorder is characterized by antisocial behavior (behaviors also common in ADHD) and persistent or consistent pattern of defiance, disobedience, and hostility toward various authority figures, including parents, teachers, and other adults.

Oppositional defiant disorder is more common in boys until after puberty, when rates become equal. The etiology is unknown but is likely due to a combination of biological, genetic, and psychosocial factors. Oppositional defiant disorder is sometimes a precursor of conduct disorder.

Conduct Disorder (CD)

Conduct disorder is characterized by antisocial behavior and may follow ODD. Behaviors include aggression with fighting, bullying, intimidating, assaulting, sexually coercing, and/or cruelty to people and/or animals. Other behaviors include vandalism, theft, truancy, early alcohol and substance abuse, and precocious sexual activity.

The etiology is unknown but is probably due to a combination of biological, genetic, and psychosocial factors. Children with chronic illness have a 2 to 5 times increased incidence of CD, especially if they have developmental or neurologic disabilities. Dysfunctional parenting, especially harsh, inconsistent, rejecting, and abusive forms, predispose to the development of CD.

Why Is It Important to Include Disruptive Disorders in History, Observation, and Surveillance?

Disruptive behavior disorders in children are common. Studies indicate that 4% to 12% of school-aged children have ADHD. The prevalence of ODD and CD is 1% to 6% of school-aged children. Symptoms can also be an indication of other problems, such as child abuse, neglect, or parental discord.

Disruptive disorders often accompany other behavioral conditions and risk behaviors. Learning disabilities, mood and anxiety disorders, and alcohol and other substance use disorders are common in children with a disruptive disorder.

The rate at which these and other mental health problems are detected is improving but is still less than ideal. Despite the prevalence of 10% to 20% in community samples and the repeated contact physicians have with young children, the treated prevalence estimates are increasing but still lower than ideal.

Early intervention has powerful benefits. Early intervention is less costly and more successful than later interventions. Early intervention also may prevent persistent dysfunctional behavior patterns from becoming established. Children with ADHD and CD who are not treated are more likely to experience drug abuse, antisocial behavior, teen pregnancy, and injuries.

Mental health screening has been recommended by national organizations. Healthy People 2010, the Surgeon General's Report on Children's Mental Health, and the President's New Freedom Commission on Mental Health all recommend pediatric mental health screening in primary care.

The US Preventive Services Task Force has not specifically evaluated the evidence regarding screening for disruptive behavior disorders.

How Should You Conduct Surveillance and Screening for Disruptive Disorders?

Surveillance is a flexible, continuous process of monitoring a child's developmental and behavioral status during health supervision visits. It also may include history-taking and the use of structured parent questionnaires.

Screening is assessing for conditions in asymptomatic patients and is part of behavioral surveillance. It includes the use of structured parent questionnaires.

Diagnosis of behavioral disorders typically occurs after surveillance and/or screening reveals concerns in one or more functional areas.

Talk With Parents

At each yearly health supervision visit of school-aged children and adolescents, conduct mental health surveillance by asking parents questions, such as

- How is your child doing in school?

- Are there any problems with learning that you or the teacher has seen?

- Is your child happy in school?

- Are you concerned with any behavioral problems in school, at home, or when your child is playing with friends?

- Is your child having problems completing class work or homework?

- Does your child mind you or follow rules as expected?

- Do you have resources to assist you (eg, family members, child care, adequate financial support)?

- How are things going at home (eg, marital problems, substance abuse, domestic violence)?

Consider a Broad-band Screening Instrument

At the 5-, 6-, and 7-year health supervision visits, consider using a broad-band screening instrument, such as the Pediatric Symptom Checklist, to assess behavior.

- If broad-band screening points toward specific problems, such as attention, hyperactivity, or oppositional behavior problems, consider using one of the "narrow-band tools" listed in the Resources section to facilitate assessment. For more information about screening tools, see the Resources section of the "Developmental and Behavioral Considerations" chapter.

- If symptoms are identified in multiple areas with the broad-band instrument, refer for full developmental and learning assessment.

What Should You Do With an Abnormal Result?

Assure parents they are not alone and that support is available if they need it. Stress that behavior disorders are treatable and that early intervention is preferable to improve long-term outlook.

Offer to initiate a referral to a mental health professional, support group, or other therapeutic agency. Initiate an immediate referral to a mental health practitioner or facility if a child shows severe impairment, such as danger to self or others.

If a specific diagnosis is made in the primary care setting, begin educating parents about the chronic nature of the condition. Provide a list of print and online resources. Help parents meet other parents and learn about other community resources, such as support groups.

Schedule frequent office visits to follow up with the family and child. If treatment will occur in the primary care office, consult the American Academy of Pediatrics ADHD clinical practice guidelines and those of the AAP Task Force on Mental Health available at: http://pediatrics. aappublications.org/content/vol125/Supplement_3.

Two Toolkits are available with forms and billing information:

- Addressing Mental Health Concerns in Primary Care: A Clinician's Toolkit (aap.org/bookstore)

- Caring for Children with ADHD: A Resource Toolkit for Clinicians (http://www.nichq.org/adhd.html)

What Results Should You Document?

Document parent and teacher questionnaires, to whom referral was made, follow-up plans, and current treatment(s).

ICD-9-CM Codes

312.xx	Disturbance of conduct (CD)
313.81	Oppositional defiant disorder (ODD)
314.xx	Attention-deficit/hyperactivity disorder (ADHD)
V71.02	Childhood or adolescent antisocial behavior
V40.3	Other behavioral problems

The American Academy of Pediatrics publishes a complete line of coding publications, including an annual edition of *Coding for Pediatrics*. For more information on these excellent resources, visit the American Academy of Pediatrics Online Bookstore at **www.aap.org/bookstore/.**

Resources

Policy and Guidelines

Achieving the Promise: Transforming Mental Health Care in America. Rockville, MD: The President's New Freedom Commission on Mental Health; 2003. http://www. mentalhealthcommission.gov/

American Academy of Pediatrics Committee on Quality Improvement. Clinical practice guideline: diagnosis and evaluation of the school-aged child with attention-deficit/ hyperactivity disorder. *Pediatrics*. 2000;105(5):1158–1170. http://aappolicy.aappublications.org/cgi/content/full/ pediatrics%3b105/5/1158

American Academy of Pediatrics Committee on Quality Improvement. Clinical practice guideline: treatment of the school-aged child with attention-deficit/ hyperactivity disorder. *Pediatrics*. 2001;108(4):1033–1044. http://aappolicy.aappublications.org/cgi/content/full/ pediatrics%3b105/5/1158

Greenhill L, Abikoff H, Arnold L, et al. *Psychopharmacological Treatment Manual, NIMH Multimodal Treatment Study of Children With Attention Deficit Hyperactivity Disorder (MTA Study)*. New York, NY: Psychopharmacology Subcommittee of the MTA Steering Committee; 1998

Institute of Medicine. *Crossing the Quality Chasm: A New Health System for the 21st Century*. Washington, DC: National Academy Press; 2000. http://www.nap.edu/ books/0309072808/html/

National Institutes of Health Consensus Statement. Diagnosis and treatment of attention deficit hyperactivity disorder (ADHD). 1998;110. http://consensus.nih.gov/1998/1998AttentionDeficitHyperactivityDisorder110html.htm

Articles

General

American Psychiatric Association. *Diagnostic and Statistical Manual of Mental Disorders.* 4th ed. Text rev. Washington, DC: American Psychiatric Association; 2000

Brown RT, Freeman WS, Perrin JM, et al. Prevalence and assessment of attention-deficit/hyperactivity disorder in primary care settings. *Pediatrics.* 2001;107(3):e43

Dey AN, Schiller JS, Tai, DA. Summary health statistics for US children: National Health Interview Survey, 2002. *Vital Health Stat.* 2004;10(221). http://www.cdc.gov/nchs/data/series/sr_10/sr10_221.pdf

Dobos AE, Dworkin PH, Bernstein BA. Pediatricians' approaches to developmental problems: has the gap been narrowed? *J Dev Behav Pediatr.* 1994;15:34–38

Kelleher KJ, Childs GE, Wasserman RC, McInerny TK, Nutting PA, Gardner WP. Insurance status and recognition of psychosocial problems: a report from PROS and ASPN. *Arch Pediatr Adolesc Med.* 1997;151:1109–1115

Kelleher KJ, Wolraich ML. Diagnosing psychosocial problems. *Pediatrics.* 1996;97:899–901

Kelleher KJ, McInerny TK, Gardner WP, Childs GE, Wasserman RC. Increasing identification of psychosocial problems: 1979–1996. *Pediatrics.* 2000;105:1313–1321

Mrazek PJ, Haggerty RJ, ed. *Reducing Risks for Mental Disorders: Frontiers for Preventive Intervention Research.* Washington, DC: Institute of Medicine National Academy Press; 1994. http://www.nap.edu/books/0309049393/html

Pavuluri MN, Luk SL, McGee R. Help-seeking for behavior problems by parents of preschool children: a community study. *J Am Acad Child Adolesc Psychiatry.* 1996;35(2):215–222

Reynolds AJ, Temple JA, Robertson DL, Mann EA. Long-term effects of an early childhood intervention on educational achievement and juvenile arrest: a 15-year follow-up of low-income children in public schools. *JAMA.* 2001;285:2339–2346

Shaffer D, Fisher P, Lucas CP, Dulcan MK, Schwab-Stone ME. NIMH Diagnostic Interview Schedule for Children Version IV (NIMH DISC-IV): description, differences from previous versions, and reliability of some common diagnoses. *J Am Acad Child Adolesc Psychiatry.* 2000;39(1):28–38

Thomas CR, Holzer CE. National distribution of child and adolescent psychiatrists. *J Am Acad Child Adolesc Psychiatry.* 1999;38:9–15

US Department of Health and Human Services. *Mental Health: A Report of the Surgeon General—Executive Summary.* Rockville, MD: US Department of Health and Human Services, Substance Abuse and Mental Health Services Administration, Center for Mental Health Services, National Institutes of Health, National Institute of Mental Health; 1999

US Department of Health and Human Services. *Report of the Surgeon General's Conference on Children's Mental Health: A National Action Agenda.* Rockville, MD: US Department of Health and Human Services; 2001. http://www.surgeongeneral.gov/library/mentalhealth/home.html

Clinical Features

Biederman J, Faraone SV. Attention-deficit hyperactivity disorder. *Lancet.* 2005;366(9481):237–248

Connor D, Edwards G, Fletcher KE, et al. Correlates of comorbid psychopathology in children with ADHD. *J Am Acad Child Adolesc Psychiatry.* 2003;42:193–200

Jensen PS, Martin D, Cantwell DP. Comorbidity in ADHD: implications for research, practice, and DSM-V. *J Am Acad Child Adolesc Psychiatry.* 1997;36(8):1065–1079

Modestin J, Matutat B, Wurmle O. Antecedents of opioid dependence and personality disorder: attention-deficit/hyperactivity disorder and conduct disorder. *Eur Arch Psychiatry Clin Neurosci.* 2001;251(1):42–47

Shaffer D, Fisher P, Dulcan MK, et al. The NIMH Diagnostic Interview Schedule for Children Version 2.3 (DISC-2.3): description, acceptability, prevalence rates, and performance in the MECA Study. Methods for the Epidemiology of Child and Adolescent Mental Disorders Study. *J Am Acad Child Adolesc Psychiatry.* 1996;35:865–877

Wilens TC, Faraone, SV, Biederman J, Gunawardene S. Does stimulant therapy of attention-deficit/hyperactivity disorder beget later substance abuse? A meta-analytic review of the literature. *Pediatrics.* 2003;111:1:179–185

Wolraich ML, Lindgren S, Stromquist A, Milich R, Davis C, Watson D. Stimulant medication use by primary care physicians in the treatment of attention deficit hyperactivity disorder. *Pediatrics.* 1990;86:95–101

Wolraich ML, Hannah JN, Pinnock TY, Baumgaertel A, Brown J. Comparison of diagnostic criteria for attention-deficit hyperactivity disorder in a county-wide sample. *J Am Acad Child Adolesc Psychiatry.* 1996; 35:319–324

Screening and Screening Tools

American Academy of Pediatrics Committee on Children With Disabilities. Developmental surveillance and screening of infants and young children. *Pediatrics.* 2001;108(1):192–195

Achenbach TM. *Manual for the Child Behavior Checklist/4–18 and 1991 Profile.* Burlington, VT: University of Vermont, Department of Psychiatry; 1991

Collett BR, Ohan JL, Myers KM. Ten-year review of rating scales. V: scales assessing attention-deficit/hyperactivity disorder. *J Am Acad Child Adolesc Psychiatry.* 2003;42(9):1015–1037

Conners CK. *Conners' Rating Scales—Revised: Instruments for Use With Children and Adolescents.* New York, NY: Multi-Health Systems, Inc; 1997

Conners C, Wells K. *Conners-Wells Adolescent Self-Report Scale.* North Tonowanda, NY: Multi-Health Systems; 1997

Duggan AK, Starfield B, DeAngelis C. Structured encounter form: the impact on provider performance and recording of well-child care. *Pediatrics.* 1990;85:104–113

Eyberg S. *Eyberg Child Behavior Inventory & Sutter-Eyberg Student Behavior Inventory-Revised (ECBI/SESBI-R).* Lutz, FL: Psychological Assessment Resources; 1999

Gardner W, Murphy M, Childs G, et al. The PSC-17: a brief pediatric symptom checklist including psychosocial problem subscales: a report from PROS and ASPN. *Ambul Child Health.* 1999;5:225–236

Glascoe FP. Parents' concerns about children's development: prescreening technique or screening test? *Pediatrics.* 1997;99:522–528

Glascoe FP, Dworkin PH. The role of parents in the detection of developmental and behavioral problems. *Pediatrics.* 1995;95:829–836

Ilfeld F. Further validation of a psychiatric symptom index in a normal population. *Psychology Rep.* 1976;39:1215–1228

Jellinek MS, Murphy JM, Robinson J, Feins A, Lamb S, Fenton T. Pediatric Symptom Checklist: screening school-age children for psychosocial dysfunction. *J Pediatr.* 1988;112:201–209

Jellinek M, Patel B, Froehle M. *Bright Futures in Practice: Mental Health Tool Kit.* Arlington, VA: National Center for Education in Maternal and Child Health; 2002

Kemper K. Self-administered questionnaire for structured psychosocial screening in pediatrics. *Pediatrics.* 1992;89:433–436

Kemper KJ, Kelleher KJ. Family psychosocial screening: instruments and techniques. *Ambul Child Health.* 1996;4:325–339

Reynolds C, Kamphaus, R. *Behavior Assessment System for Children.* 2nd Edition. Shoreview, MN: AGS Publishing; 1998

Books for Parents

Barkley R. *Taking Charge of ADHD: The Complete Authoritative Guide for Parents.* New York, NY: The Guilford Press; 2000

Brazelton TB. *Touchpoints: Three to Six: Your Child's Emotional and Behavioral Development.* Cambridge, MA: Perseus Publishing; 2002

Glasser H, Easley J. *Transforming the Difficult Child, The Nurtured Heart Approach.* Tucson, AZ: Nurtured Heart Publications; 1999

Greene RW. *The Explosive Child: A New Approach for Understanding and Parenting Easily Frustrated, Chronically Inflexible Children.* New York, NY: HarperCollins Publishers; 1998

Riley D. *The Defiant Child : A Parent's Guide to Oppositional Defiant Disorder.* Dallas, TX: Taylor Publishing Company; 1997

Turecki S. *The Difficult Child.* Rev ed. New York City, NY: Bantam; 1989

Broad-band Screening Scales and Tools

Broad-band tools assess a relatively full range of behavioral and emotional symptoms and disorders.

Pediatric Symptom Checklist

http://www2.massgeneral.org/allpsych/psc/psc_home.htm

Developed to facilitate recognition and referral of child psychosocial problems by primary care pediatricians

- 35-item parent report and 35-item youth self-report (awailable free online)

- Spanish versions of both and a Japanese parent report available

- A brief 17-item parent-report in English available (not available online)

- Overall sum represents parental impression of their child's psychosocial functioning

- Discrete subscales for attentional, oppositional, and internalizing symptoms

- Strong internal consistency, test-retest reliability, and validity with psychiatric assessments of child functioning

Behavior Assessment System for Children, 2nd Edition—BASC-2

http://www.pearsonassessments.com/HAIWEB/Cultures/en-us/Productdetail.htm?Pid=PAa30000

Available for purchase

- 100- to 150-item (number of items vary depending on child's age) parent report of competencies and problem behaviors

- Spanish version available

- Teacher and youth self-reports available

- Discrete subscales for attentional, oppositional, and internalizing symptoms

- Strong internal consistency, test-retest reliability, and validity with psychiatric assessments of child functioning

- Recently updated

Child Behavior Checklist—CBCL

http://www.aseba.org/ Available for purchase

- 118-item parent report of competencies and problem behaviors

- Spanish version available

- Teacher and youth self-reports also available

- Discrete subscales for attentional, oppositional, and internalizing symptoms

- Recently updated with new normative data

Conners Rating Scales-Revised—CRS-R

http://psychcorp.pearsonassessments.com/HAIWEB/Cultures/en-us/Productdetail.htm?Pid=PAg116

Available for purchase

- First developed in 1970 to assess a wide variety of children's common behavior problems, such as sleep disturbance, eating problems, and peer relationships

- CRS-R includes items specific to *DSM-IV*–defined ADHD and its associated features and updates age and gender normative values

- Parent and teacher forms available in full (80-item, 59-item) and abbreviated (27-item, 28-item) versions

- Adolescent self-report (Conners-Wells' Adolescent Self-Report Scale) in full and abbreviated versions also available

Narrow-band Screening Scales and Tools

Narrow-band tools assess specific diagnostic categories.

NICHQ-Vanderbilt ADHD Rating Scales
Parents' scale

http://www.pedialliance.com/forms/ADHD_Parent_Assessment41.pdf

Teacher's scale

http://www.brightfutures.org/mentalhealth/pdf/professionals/bridges/adhd.pdf

- Both scales available free online

- Assess for symptom presence and severity in school, home, and social settings based on *DSM-IV* diagnostic criteria

No specific tools have been scientifically validated for screening in the pediatric practice. However, several screening tools have been shown to be effective when implemented in primary care pediatric offices.

Screening Questions for IPV

Use the 4-question "Child Safety Questionnaire."[1]

- Have you ever been in a relationship with someone who has hit you, kicked you, slapped you, punched you, or threatened to hurt you?

- Are you currently in a relationship with someone who has hit you, kicked you, slapped you, punched you, sexually abused you, or threatened to hurt you?

- When you were pregnant did anyone ever physically hurt you?

- Are you in a relationship with someone who yells at you, calls you names, or puts you down?

What Should You Do if You Identify IPV?

The pediatricians' job is not to fix the problem but to

- Provide a safe environment for disclosure and discussion of the issue.

- Support the victim.

- Begin to help the victim understand her situation and to educate and address the impact of IPV on her children.

The key is to assess for safety and report IPV if it is mandated. If you identify IPV,

- Provide referrals to social workers; local IPV support groups; or shelters, mental health or counseling, or legal services.

- Document the problem so that other practitioners will be aware of any disclosure, but develop a protocol for confidentiality because the perpetrator may have access to a child's records.

- If you need to report to child protective services, inform the mother, assess for possible increase in violence, and arrange a safe place for the woman and her children to go.

Understanding the dynamics of IPV is key to successful support and intervention. Women may not disclose violence, but through surveillance and screening you can help them be aware that this is an important issue they can discuss with you when ready. Many women do not leave violent relationships for a variety of reasons, but you can still help them keep their children and themselves safer.

What Results Should You Document?

Documentation requirements and laws may vary by state and locality. The documentation described below is suggested based on methods used in Rochester, NY, as of 2008.

If perpetrator has no access to patient's chart

- Use the patient's (or injured's) own words regarding injury and abuse.

- For injured patients, legibly document all injuries. Use a body map and take photographs of injuries, if possible.

If perpetrator does or may have access to child's chart, or uncertain

- Use charting phrases that you have dedicated exclusively to IPV, such as

  ▸ "Family concerns discussed" for screening done

  ▸ "Resources offered" for positive screens

ICD-9-CM Codes	
E960–E969	Homicide and injury purposely inflicted by other persons
E967	Child battering and other maltreatment
E967.0	by parent
308	Acute reaction to stress
308.4	Mixed disorders as reaction to stress
308.9	Unspecified acute reaction to stress

The American Academy of Pediatrics publishes a complete line of coding publications, including an annual edition of *Coding for Pediatrics*. For more information on these excellent resources, visit the American Academy of Pediatrics Online Bookstore at **www.aap.org/bookstore/**.

Sample Screening Card

(available for reproduction and distribution to office staff)

Intimate Partner Violence: Have You Screened Today?

What is intimate partner violence?

Abuse in relationships, including pushing, shoving, slapping, punching, choking, kicking, holding, tying down, assault with a weapon, and economic/emotional isolation.

How big is this problem?

- Police in the United States spend one-third of their time responding to domestic violence calls.

- It is estimated that 2 million women are assaulted by their partners each year in the United States. This is the major source of injury to women 14 to 45 years old, causing more injuries than accidents, muggings, and rapes combined.

Why do we need to ask?

- Intimate partner violence against mothers is a pediatric issue.

- The American Academy of Pediatrics recommends pediatricians attempt to recognize evidence of family violence and intervene to maximize safety.

- Between 50% and 70% of men who abuse female partners also physically abuse children.

- Children that witness intimate partner violence show such symptoms as stuttering, bedwetting, insomnia, separation anxiety, difficulty concentrating, headaches, abdominal pain, and aggressive behavior.

Why don't we ask?

- Fear of offending

- Lack of time

- Discomfort with the subject

- Biases about who is affected (ie, socioeconomic status, race, age, education, marital status [none of which matter])

- Inability to give a solution

How can we ask?

With anticipatory guidance

If "Yes"

- Validate.

- Listen nonjudgmentally.

- Encourage communication.

- Reassure them your office is a safe place to talk and find information.

- Refer them to the appropriate resources.

If "No"

- They are now aware your office is a safe place to talk and to receive information.

- They know that you are concerned and willing to talk about this subject.

1. Be direct in your questioning.

2. - "I ask all my patients this question because I want you to know this is a safe place where help is available. Your health and well-being are important to me and may affect your children's safety and well-being."

   - "Because violence is so common, I have started to routinely ask all of my patients about violence in the home."

3. - "Are you in a relationship where you are being hurt physically or emotionally?"

   - "Have you ever been emotionally or physically abused by your partner? By this I mean have you ever been hit, kicked, slapped, punched, or isolated from your family or someone important to you by your partner?"

Stalking

While Bright Futures does not provide specific guidance on discussing or counseling on stalking, the general prevalence and ties to IPV deserve a mention for practitioners to build awareness. Stalking is a common problem in the United States. It affects 1 in 12 women and 1 in 45 men at some time during their lives. In a national study of college students, 13% of college women report having been stalked.

Most of those who are stalked know their stalker because they had a personal or romantic relationship before the stalking behavior began. The stalkers may be classmates, coworkers, friends, or former girlfriends or boyfriends.

Although many people do not report being stalked, this behavior is unpredictable and serious, and can become violent over time. In fact, 3 out of 4 women killed by an intimate partner were stalked by their killer in the year before their murder.

Stalking

The legal definition of stalking varies by jurisdiction, but it is generally considered an action or conduct by a person that makes a reasonable person feel afraid or in danger. Stalking is considered a crime in all 50 states. Stalking behaviors include

- Showing up at places uninvited
- Watching from afar
- Following
- Repeatedly calling, e-mailing, and text messaging
- Sending letters or gifts
- Contacting family or friends

For individuals being stalked, provide the following recommendations:

- Trust your instincts.
- Do not attempt to communicate with your stalker.
- Tell someone.
- Keep records of calls, e-mails, or other communications as evidence.

- Contact local service hotlines and police.
- Obtain a protection order.

Screening Questions for Stalking

Has anyone phoned, paged, written, e-mailed, followed, or watched you or attempted contact with you in other ways that made you afraid or concerned for your safety?

Resources

Policy and Evidence-based Guidelines

American Academy of Pediatrics Committee on Child Abuse and Neglect. The role of the pediatrician in recognizing and intervening on behalf of abused women. *Pediatrics.* 1998;101:1091–1092

Intimate Partner Violence and Healthy People 2010 Fact Sheet. Family Violence Prevention Fund. http://endabuse.org/userfiles/file/HealthCare/healthy_people_2010.pdf

US Advisory Board on Child Abuse and Neglect. *A Nation's Shame: Fatal Child Abuse and Neglect in the United States.* Washington, DC: US Department of Health and Human Services. 1995. http://ican-ncfr.org/documents/Nations-Shame.pdf

US Department of Health and Human Services. Office of Disease Prevention and Health Promotion. http://www.healthypeople.gov

Screening Tools

American Medical Association. Diagnostic and treatment guidelines on domestic violence. *Arch Fam Med.* 1992;1(1):39–47

Groves B, Augustyn M, Lee D, Sawires P. *Identifying and Responding to Domestic Violence: Consensus Recommendations for Child and Adolescent Health.* San Francisco, CA: Family Violence Prevention Fund; 2002

Nelson HD. Screening for domestic violence—bridging the evidence gaps. *Lancet.* 2004;364(suppl 1):S22–S23

Parkinson GW, Adams RC, Emerling FG. Maternal domestic violence screening in an office-based pediatric practice. *Pediatrics.* 2001;108:e43

Rennison CM. *Intimate Partner Violence, 1993–2001.* Washington, DC: US Department of Justice Bureau of Justice Statistics; 2003

Siegel RM, Hill TD, Henderson VA, Ernst HM, Boat BW. Screening for IPV in the community pediatric setting. *Pediatrics*. 1999;104:874–877

Wahl RA, Sisk DJ, Ball TM. Clinic-based screening for domestic violence: use of a child safety questionnaire. *BMC Med*. 2004;2:25

Articles

Augustyn M, Groves BM. If we don't ask, they aren't going to tell: screening for domestic violence. *Contemp Pediatr*. 2005;22(9):43–50

Erickson MJ, Hill TD, Siegel RM. Barriers to domestic violence screening in the pediatric setting. *Pediatrics*. 2001;108(1):98–102

Fisher BS, Cullen FT, Turner MG. *Sexual Victimization of College Women*. Washington, DC: US Department of Justice, National Institute of Justice: December 2000. http://www.ncjrs.gov/txtfiles1/nij/182369.txt

Greenfeld LA, Rand MR, Craven D, et al. *Violence by Intimates: Analysis of Data on Crimes by Current or Former Spouses, Boyfriends, and Girlfriends*. Washington, DC: US Department of Justice; 1998. http://www.ojp.usdoj.gov/bjs/pub/pdf/vi.pdf[

Huth-Bocks AC, Levendosky AA, Bogat GA. The effects of domestic violence during pregnancy on maternal and infant health. *Violence Vict*. 2002;17(2):169–185

Knapp JF, Dowd MD. Family violence: implications for the pediatrician. *Pediatr Rev*. 1998;19:316

McFarlane JM, Campbell JC, Wilt S, et al. Stalking and intimate partner femicide. *Homicide Studies*. 1999;3(4):300–316

Parker B, McFarlane J, Soeken K. Abuse during pregnancy: effects on maternal complications and birth weight in adult and teenage women. *Obstet Gynecol*. 1994;84(3):323–328

Parkinson GW, Adams RC, Emerling FG. Maternal domestic violence screening in an office-based pediatric practice. *Pediatrics*. 2001;108:e43

Rennison C. *Intimate Partner Violence, Special Report 1993–2000*. Washington, DC: Bureau of Justice Statistics, US Department of Justice; 2000. Publication No. NCJ178247

Siegel RM, Hill TD, Henderson VA, Ernst HM, Boat BW. Screening for IPV in the community pediatric setting. *Pediatrics*. 1999;104:874–877

Silverman JG, Raj A, Mucci LA, Hathaway JE. Dating violence against adolescent girls and associated substance use, unhealthy weight control, sexual risk behavior, pregnancy, and suicidality. *JAMA*. 2001;286(5):572–579

Tjaden P, Thoennes N. *Extent, Nature, and Consequences of Intimate Partner Violence: Findings From the National Violence Against Women Survey*. Washington, DC: National Institute of Justice, Centers for Disease Control and Prevention; 2000. http://www.ojp.usdoj.gov/nij/pubs-sum/181867.htm.

Tjaden P, Thoennes N. *Full Report of the Prevalence, Incidence, and Consequences of Violence Against Women: Findings From the National Violence Against Women Survey*. Washington, DC: US Department of Justice, National Institute of Justice, Centers for Disease Control and Prevention; 2000. http://www.ncjrs.org/txtfiles1/nij/183781.txt

Tjaden P, Thoennes N. *Stalking in America: Findings From the National Violence Against Women Survey*. Washington, DC: US Department of Justice, National Institute of Justice and Centers for Disease Control and Prevention; 1998

Zuckerman BS, Beardslee WR. Maternal depression: a concern for pediatricians. *Pediatrics*. 1987;79:110–117

Web Sites for Physicians' Offices

LEAP (Look to End Abuse Permanently), http://leapsf.org/html/index.shtml An organization of healthcare providers and volunteers dedicated to ending intimate partner violence and family violence by establishing screening, treatment, and prevention programs in the health care setting.

Identifying and Responding to Domestic Violence: Consensus Recommendations for Child and Adolescent Health:
(1) http://endabuse.org/section/programs/children_families/_description
(2) http://www.endabuse.org/userfiles/file/HealthCare/pediatric.pdf
Developed by the Family Violence Prevention Fund's National Health Resource Center on Domestic Violence, these recommendations are the first of their kind to

address how to assess children and youth for domestic violence, and specifically offer recommendations on assessing adults for victimization with children present.

Violence against Women Online Resources:
http://www.vaw.umn.edu/categories/I,II
This site provides materials on domestic violence, sexual assault, and stalking for criminal justice professionals, sexual assault and domestic violence victim advocates, and other multidisciplinary professionals and community partners who respond to these crimes.

Web Sites for National Organizations

Family Violence Prevention Fund (FVPF):
http://endabuse.org/
FVPF develops strategies, programs, and resources to stop family violence. Its Web site offers a news desk and prevention toolkits and information on FVPF programs and services in public education, child welfare, immigration, public health, and criminal justice.

Institute on Violence Abuse and Trauma:
www.ivatcenters.org
The institute provides information, networking, training, education, and program evaluation for other agencies, practitioners, and organizations. Provides information on many areas of family violence and sexual assault, maintains a clearinghouse, and publishes a quarterly bulletin.

National Center on Domestic and Sexual Violence
http://www.ncdsv.org/ncd_about.html
This organization helps a myriad of professionals who work with victims and perpetrators; law enforcement; criminal justice professionals such as prosecutors, judges and probation officers; health care professionals including emergency response teams, nurses and doctors; domestic violence and sexual assault advocates and service providers; and counselors and social workers. In addition to these professionals, NCDSV also works with local, state and federal agencies; state and national organizations; educators, researchers, faith community leaders, media community leaders, elected officials, policymakers and others.

National Coalition Against Domestic Violence (NCADV):
http://www.ncadv.org/aboutus.php
The mission of NCADV is to work for major societal changes necessary to eliminate both personal and

societal violence against all women and children. This site provides general IPV resources, statistics, action alerts, and materials for victims, including safety plans and protecting your identity.

National Violence Against Women Prevention Research Center (NVAWPRC):
http://www.musc.edu/vawprevention/
Sponsored by the Centers for Disease Control and Prevention, this Web site is designed to be useful to scientists, practitioners, IPV advocates, grassroots organizations, and any other professional or layperson interested in current topics related to violence against women and its prevention.

Office on Violence Against Women
http://www.ovw.usdoj.gov/
Office on Violence Against Women (OVW) at the U.S. Department of Justice administers financial and technical assistance to communities across the country that are developing programs, policies, and practices aimed at ending domestic violence, dating violence, sexual assault, and stalking.

Web Sites for Adolescents

PromoteTruth.org
Promote Truth provides support and information about sexual violence issues for teens and their communities. Their Web site offers information and online services, including anonymous use of message boards for targeted audiences: teens, parents, teachers, and other professionals.

LoveisRespect.org/
This Web site provides resources for teens, parents, friends and family, peer advocates, government officials, law enforcement officials, and the general public. All communication is confidential and anonymous.

National Teen Dating Abuse Helpline
Launched in February 2007 with help from founding sponsor Liz Claiborne Inc. It is a national 24-hour resource that can be accessed by phone or the Internet and specifically designed for teens and young adults. The helpline and loveisrespect.org offer real-time one-on-one support from trained Peer Advocates. Managed by the National Domestic Violence Hotline, loveisrespect, National Teen Dating Abuse Helpline operates from a call center in Austin, TX. Peer advocates are trained to offer support, information, and advocacy to those involved in

dating abuse relationships as well as concerned parents, teachers, clergy, law enforcement, and service providers.

866/331-9474 | 866/331-8453 TTY

SeeitandStopit.org
Public awareness Web site, maintained by the Teen Action Campaign, offers facts, statistics, and testimony on teen dating violence and provides information on how teens can get help for themselves or a friend and a toolkit for starting a school organization.

Web Sites for Victims

Call to Protect:
http://www.wirelessfoundation.org/CalltoProtect/index.cfm
This program distributes wireless phones to help combat domestic violence. The program is a national initiative of the wireless industry and NCADV.

Domestic Violence: National Directory of Professional Services:
http://www.soros.org/initiatives/justice
This online directory is an interactive resource that offers contact information for agencies providing services to victims, batterers, or their families. The interactive feature allows users to seek assistance directly from the desktop while browsing the material online.

National Domestic Violence Hotline:
http://www.ndvh.org/

800/799-SAFE (800/799-7233)

TTY: 800/787-3224

Staff provides callers with crisis intervention, information about domestic violence, and referrals to local programs 24 hours a day, 7 days a week. Telephone assistance is available in many languages, including Spanish.

Office for Victims of Crime (OVC):
http://www.ojp.usdoj.gov/ovc/help/dv.htm#l
Established by the 1984 Victims of Crime Act to oversee diverse programs that benefit victims of crime. The OVC provides substantial funding to state victim assistance and compensation programs.

Social Security Administration—Domestic Violence:
http://www.ssa.gov/pressoffice/domestic_fact.html
The division instructs victims of domestic violence on how to apply for a new Social Security number.

Witness Justice:
http://www.witnessjustice.org/
Witness Justice provides trauma victims and their families with resources that promote physical, psychological, and spiritual healing. The site features access to experts, message boards, and other print and electronic victim resources.

Helpline and Web Sites on Stalking
800-FYI-CALL for assistance related to stalking.

Stalking Resource Center:
www.ncvc.org/src
A continually growing resource for practitioners and victims, the Stalking Resource Center Web site provides diverse resources, including fact sheets on federal statutes, an annotated stalking bibliography, summaries of state stalking laws, a guide to online resources, statistical overviews, practitioner profiles, and more.

Violence Against Women
This specialty page will provide you with information on all types of violence against women, including specific resources and information on how to get help.
http://www.womenshealth.gov/violence/

Reference

1. Wahl RA, Sisk DJ, Ball TM. Clinic-based screening for domestic violence: use of a child safety questionnaire. *BMC Medicine*. 2004;30(2):25

AMY HENEGHAN, MD

MATERNAL DEPRESSION

In the Bright Futures Guidelines, maternal depression is a priority for anticipatory guidance at the 1-month and 2-month visits, and Bright Futures encourages assessing for maternal depression at the 1-, 2-, and 6-month visits. Given that maternal depression can appear at any time, a sensitive and open approach to identifying and discussing maternal depression in health supervision care is warranted.

What Is Maternal Depression?

Maternal depression describes chronic or acutely depressed women with dependent children. A spectrum of diseases and disease severities exist within maternal depression, including postpartum blues, perinatal depression, postpartum depression, and postpartum psychosis.

Postpartum blues occurs in approximately 70% of women, lasts about 10 days, and typically does not interfere with a woman's ability to function.

Postpartum depression is more persistent and debilitating than postpartum blues. It occurs in approximately 15% of women, may develop insidiously over the first 3 postpartum months or more acutely, and lasts an average of 7 months if left untreated.

Postpartum depression is considered the most common complication of childbearing. Of 4 million births annually, it affects 500,000 women. It often interferes with the mother's ability to care for herself or her child.

The signs and symptoms of postpartum depression are clinically indistinguishable from major depression that occurs in women at other times. They include

- Feeling of sadness or low mood, feeling "down," feeling worthless

- Loss of interest and/or pleasure in usual activities

- Excessive or inappropriate guilt

- General fatigue and loss of energy

- Thoughts of death

- Anxiety, including worries or obsessions about the infant's health and well-being. The mother may have ambivalent or negative feelings toward the infant. She may also have intrusive and unpleasant fears or thoughts about harming the infant.

Postpartum psychosis occurs in 1 to 2 of every 1,000 births and presents within the first 2 weeks of delivery. It is characterized by the acute onset of major disturbances in thinking and behavior, hallucinations, and delusions. It is a psychiatric emergency requiring immediate action because of the risk of suicide and infanticide.

Why Is It Important to Include Maternal Depression in History, Observation, and Surveillance?

Maternal depression is a common and serious problem. Depression is the leading cause of disease burden worldwide among women ages 15 to 44. Epidemiologic and clinical studies suggest that 8% to 12% of mothers may experience postpartum depression, and elevated depressive symptoms may be present in 24% of mothers.

Maternal depression occurs in 10% to 15% of women in the general population. Rates of depressive *symptoms* are reported in 12% to 42%.

It likely has multiple causes. Although the causes of maternal depression are still unclear, it may involve a complex interaction of biochemical, interpersonal, and social factors.

Many women are at risk of developing maternal depression. Women at highest risk are those with a personal or family history of depression, a previous episode of postpartum depression, low income, low level of education, poor maternal health status, or other stressful life events.

It has serious effects on children. Numerous studies over the past 2 decades confirm that maternal depression has negative consequences for children across all ages in crucial areas, such as bonding and emotional development, behavior, mental health, and early brain development. This places a child's healthy development, especially social-emotional development, in potential peril. Thus it is imperative that the mother receive treatment to encourage the child's most optimal development.

Numerous groups have recognized it as a serious health concern and some urge action in primary care settings. Healthy People 2010 identifies depression as one of the 10 most important health concerns in the Unites States. The President's New Freedom Commission on Mental Health Report confirms that "mental illnesses rank first among illnesses that cause disability in the United States, Canada, and Western Europe" and pose "a serious public health challenge that is under-recognized as a public health burden."[1]

Depression has been highlighted by the Agency for Healthcare Research and Quality (AHRQ) and the US Preventive Services Task Force (USPSTF) as needing improved delivery of care. After an extensive review of the research evidence, AHRQ concluded that "good evidence" exists to recommend screening for depression in primary care settings.

How Should You Screen?

Use Informal Methods

- Ask questions, but not simply, "How are you doing?" Be specific in your questions.

  ▸ The USPSTF recommends 2 questions for brief maternal depression screening:

    During the past two weeks, have you ever felt down, depressed, or hopeless?

    During the past two weeks, have you felt little interest or pleasure in doing things?

  ▸ Ask about suicidal ideation.

  ▸ Ask about resources for support and assistance (eg, family members, child care, financial assistance).

  ▸ Ask about history of depression.

  ▸ Ask about other stressors that may have a negative impact (eg, marital problems, substance abuse, domestic abuse).

- Note interactions between the mother and her child.

- Listen. Mothers will talk about their concerns if they feel you are listening without judgment.

- Assure mothers that they are not alone and that there is support if they need it.

- Help mothers meet other mothers and learn about other community resources (eg, support groups).

- Encourage mothers to get the help they might need to be the best mother they can be.

Use Screening Tools

Consider using a standardized screening tool to assess a mother's symptoms. Several formal screening tools exist.

Edinburgh Postpartum Depression Scale (EPDS)

- 10-item questionnaire
- Effective and easy to use
- High scores predict mothers with depression

- In 2 large community-based studies of women up to 12 weeks postpartum, the EPDS had a sensitivity of 93% to 100% and a specificity of 83% to 90% for major depression using a cut-off score of 10 when compared to structured diagnostic interviews.

Other Helpful Depression Screening Tools

- Patient Health Questionnaire (PHQ-2 and PHQ-9)

- Center for Epidemiological Studies Depression Scale (CES-D)

- Beck Depression Inventory (BDI)

- Parenting Stress Index (PSI)

What Should You Do With an Abnormal Result?

Ask whether the mother has a primary care practitioner of her own and gain permission to initiate a conversation with that professional.

Offer to initiate a referral to a mental health professional, support group, or other therapeutic agency. Initiate an immediate referral if the mother shows severe impairment, psychosis, or suicidal ideation. If the depression is significant or prolonged, it may not be sufficient to only refer the mother for therapy. The mother-infant dyad may also need intervention for attachment concerns, in these cases referral to an Early Intervention Program may be appropriate.

Ask to speak with other family members who might be supportive to the mother and provide a list of print and online resources that might be helpful to the mother at risk.

Stress that depression is treatable. Schedule frequent office visits to follow up with the mother and her child(ren).

ICD-9-CM Codes	
296.2x	Major depressive episode
300.4	Dysthymic disorder
309.0	Adjustment disorder with mixed anxiety and depressed mood
296.2x or 296.3x	Postpartum depression
296.x4	Mood disorder with psychotic features

The American Academy of Pediatrics publishes a complete line of coding publications, including an annual edition of *Coding for Pediatrics*. For more information on these excellent resources, visit the American Academy of Pediatrics Online Bookstore at **www.aap.org/bookstore/.**

What Results Should You Document?

Record the EPDS score, the health care professional to whom any referral was made, follow-up plans (for both the mother and the child), and current treatment(s).

Resources

Evidence-based Guidelines

Committee on Quality of Health Care in America. *Crossing the Quality Chasm: A New Health System for the 21st Century.* Washington, DC: National Academy Press; 2000

Gaynes B, Gavin N, Meltzer-Brody S, et al. Perinatal depression: prevalence, screening accuracy, and screening outcomes. *Evid Rep Technol Assess (Summ).* 2005;(119):1–8

Pignone MP, Gaynes BN, Rushton JL, et al. Screening for depression in adults: a summary of the evidence for the US Preventive Services Task Force. *Ann Intern Med.* 2002;136:765–776

US Preventive Services Task Force. Screening for depression recommendations and rationale. *Ann Intern Med.* 2002;136:760–764

Books

Beardslee WR. *Out of the Darkened Room: When a Parent is Depressed: Protecting the Children and Strengthening the Family.* Boston, MA: Little Brown; 2002

Bennett S, Indman P. *Beyond the Blues: A Guide to Understanding and Treating Prenatal and Postpartum Depression.* San Jose, CA: MoodSwings Press; 2003

Goodman SH, Gotlib IH, eds. *Children of Depressed Parents: Mechanisms of Risk and Implications for Treatment.* Washington, DC: American Psychological Association; 2001

Henry AD, Clayfield JC, Phillips SM. *Parenting Well When You're Depressed: A Complete Resource for Maintaining a Healthy Family.* Oakland, CA: New Harbinger Publications; 2001

Honikman J. *I'm Listening: A Guide to Supporting Postpartum Families* Available at www.janehonikman.com/buy.html

Articles

General

President's New Freedom Commission on Mental Health. *Achieving the Promise: Transforming Mental Health Care in America. Final Report.* Rockville, MD: President's New Freedom Commission on Mental Health; 2003. DHHS Publication No. SMA-03-3832

Chaudron LH. Postpartum depression: what pediatricians need to know. *Pediatr Rev.* 2003;24:154–161

Chaudron LH, Szilagyi PG, Kitzman HJ, Wadkins HI, Conwell Y. Detection of postpartum depressive symptoms by screening at well-child visits. *Pediatrics.* 2004;113:551–558

Field T. Early intervention for infants of depressed mothers. *Pediatrics.* 1998;102:1305–1310

Frankel KA, Harmon RJ. Depressed mothers: they don't always look as bad as they feel. *J Am Acad Child Adolesc Psychiatry.* 1996;35:289–298

Heneghan AM, Silver EJ, Bauman LJ, Stein R. Do pediatricians recognize mothers with depressive symptoms? *Pediatrics.* 2000;106:1367–1373

Klinkman MS, Schwenk TL, Coyne JC. Depression in primary care—more like asthma than appendicitis: the Michigan Depression Project. Can *J Psychiatr.* 1997;42:966–973

Wisner KL, Parry BL, Pointek CM. Clinical practice. Postpartum depression. *N Engl J Med.* 2002;347:194–199

Zuckerman BS, Beardslee WR. Maternal depression: a concern for pediatricians. *Pediatrics.* 1987;79:110–117

Effects of Depression on Children

Beck CT. The effects of postpartum depression on child development: a meta-analysis. *Arch Psychiatr Nurs.* 1998;12:12–20

Goodman SH, Gotlib IH. *Children of Depressed Parents: Mechanisms of Risk and Implications for Treatment.* Washington, DC: American Psychological Association; 2001:351

McLennan JD, Offord DR. Should postpartum depression be targeted to improve child mental health? *J Am Acad Child Adolesc Psychiatry.* 2002;41:28–35

Tools

Beck AT, Ward CH, Mendelson M, Mock J, Erbaugh J. An inventory for measuring depression. *Arch Gen Psychiatry.* 1961;4:561–571

Evins GC, Theofrastous JP, Galvin SL. Postpartum depression: a comparison of screening and routine clinical evaluation. *Am J Obstet Gynecol.* 2000;182:1080–1082

Ilfeld FW. Further validation of a psychiatric symptom index in a normal population. *Psychol Rep.*1976;39:1215–1228

Jellinek M, Patel BP, Froehle MC. *Bright Futures in Practice: Mental Health Tool Kit Volume II.* Arlington, VA: National Center for Education in Maternal and Child Health; 2002

Kemper KJ. Self-administered questionnaire for structured psychosocial screening in pediatrics. *Pediatrics.* 1992;89:433–436

Kemper KJ, Babonis TR. Screening for maternal depression in pediatric clinics. *Am J Dis Child.* 1992;146:876–878

Pignone M, Gaynes BN, Rushton JL, et al. *Screening for Depression. Systematic Evidence Review No. 6.* Rockville, MD: Agency for Healthcare Research and Quality; 2002. AHRQ Publication No. 02-S002

Radloff LS. The CES-D Scale: a self report depression scale for research in the general population. *Appl Psychol Measurement.* 1977;1:385–401

Tam LW, Newton RP, Dern M, Parry BL. Screening women for postpartum depression at well baby visits: resistance encountered and recommendations. *Arch Womens Ment Health.* 2002;5:79–82

Single Item Literacy Screener (SILS) is a subjective assessment that asks patients a single question: "How often do you need to have someone help you read instructions, pamphlets, or other written material from your doctor or pharmacy?" Patients are asked to respond in terms of a 5-point Likert scale. Such screens may prove helpful in clinical practice and can be administered over the phone.

Research is lacking that might guide how best to use literacy screening in clinical practice. Be sensitive to the shame associated with low literacy, and use care in how this information is recorded on a patient's chart. Special care is needed in training environments, where care practitioners at all levels of training and experience may have access to a patient's charts.

It is not known how documentation of parental literacy in a child's medical record may be used in determining child custody, as adequacy of parental caregiving is often a point of contention in custody battles.

What Should You Do to Address Low Literacy?

Screening is not the solution, and the role of literacy screening has yet to be determined.

Health care professionals need to slow down when giving information and instructions and use a "teach-back" technique to confirm parent understanding. Avoid jargon, use plain language, and limit information to 3 to 4 key points. Communication is improved when the focus is on what parents need to know and do to best care for their child and understand why it is in their child's best interest. Using pictures and writing brief take-home information also may be helpful.

All patients benefit when health information is made easier to understand. The average US adult reads on a seventh- to eighth-grade level, while health materials are often written on a high school level, and key messages are often buried. Most patient education materials are unnecessarily complicated and based on a medical model, rather than being patient-centered. Ideally, these materials should be written to a fifth- to eighth-grade level and be formatted for reading ease.

When asking parents to teach back or "show me," providers assume responsibility for clear communication. Ask, "Can you show me how you're going to give

this medication to your son when you get home? I want to make sure I did a good job explaining this to you." The teach-back method not only can uncover misunderstanding, but also can reveal the nature of the misunderstanding and thereby allow for corrective, tailored communication.

Before literacy screening becomes part of routine care, it needs to be determined if screening and identifying patients with poor literacy and poor health literacy has an effect on practitioner-patient relationships or improves patient outcomes. Similarly, interventions to mitigate the impact of low literacy need to be tested.

For now, pediatric health care providers need to recognize the widespread nature of health literacy issues and focus on improving health communication for all patients.

Resources

Books

Doak CC, Doak LG, Root JH. *Teaching Patients with Low-Literacy Skills*. 2nd ed. Philadelphia, PA: Lippincott Williams & Wilkins; 1996

US Department of Education Institute of Education Sciences. *National Assessment of Adult Literacy (NAAL)*. Washington, DC: US Department of Education; 2003

Nielsen-Bohlman L, Panzer AM, Kindig DA. *Health Literacy: A Prescription to End Confusion*. Washington, DC: National Academies Press; 2004

Schwartzberg JG, VanGeest JB, Wang C. *Understanding Health Literacy: Implications for Medicine and Public Health*. Chicago, IL: American Medical Association Press; 2004

US Department of Health and Human Services Office of Disease Prevention and Health Promotion. *National Action Plan to Improve Health Literacy*. Washington, DC: US Department of Health and Human Services, Office of Disease Prevention and Health Promotion; 2010

Weiss BD. *Health Literacy and Patient Safety: Help Patients Understand. Manual For Clinicians*. 2nd ed. Chicago, IL: American Medical Association Foundation; 2007. http://www.ama-assn.org/ama1/pub/upload/mm/367/healthlitclinicians.pdf. (Includes strategies to enhance patient's health literacy and improve communication with patients, creating patient-friendly written materials.)

Articles

Arnold CL, Davis TC, Humiston SG, et al. Infant hearing screening: stakeholder recommendations for parent-centered communication. *Pediatrics*. 2006;117;341–354

Arnold CL, Davis TC, Ohene Frempong J, et al. Assessment of newborn screening parent education materials. *Pediatrics*. 2006;117:320–325

Berkule SB, Dreyer BP, Klass PE, Huberman HS, Yin HS, Mendelsohn AL. Mothers' expectations for shared reading after delivery: implications for reading activities at 6 months. *Ambul Pediatr*. 2008;8(3):169–174

Davis TC, Humiston SG, Arnold CL, et al. Recommendations for effective newborn screening communication: results of focus groups with parents, providers, and experts. *Pediatrics*. 2006;117:326–340

Davis TC, Wolf MS, Bass PF, et al. To err is human: literacy and misunderstanding of prescription drug labels. *Ann Intern Med*. 2006;145(12):887–894

Dewalt DA, Berkman ND, Sheridan S, Lohr KN, Pignone MP. Literacy and health outcomes: a systematic review of the literature. *J Gen Intern Med*. 2004;19(12):1228–1239

DeWalt DA, Dilling MH, Rosenthal MS, et al. Low parental literacy is associated with worse asthma care measures in children. *Ambul Pediatr*. 2007;7:25–31

Huizinga MM, Pont S, Rothman RL, Perrin E, Sanders L, Beech B. ABC's and 123's: parental literacy, numeracy, and childhood obesity. *Obes Manag*. 2008;4(3):98–103

Lokker N, Sanders L, Perrin EM, et al. Parental misinterpretations of over-the-counter pediatric cough and cold medication labels. *Pediatrics*. 2009;123(6):1464–1471

Mulvaney SA, Rothman RL, Wallston KA, Lybarger C, Dietrich MS. An internet-based program to improve self-management in adolescents with type 1 diabetes. *Diabetes Care*. 2010;33(3):602–604

Oettinger MD, Finkle JP, Esserman D, et al. Color-coding improves parental understanding of body mass index charting. *Acad Pediatr*. 2009;9(5):330–338

Parikh NS, Parker RM, Nurss JR, Baker DW, Williams MV. Shame and health literacy: the unspoken connection. *Patient Educ Couns*. 1996;27:33–39

Sanders LM, Federico S, Klass P, Abrams MA, Dreyer B. Literacy and child health: a systematic review. *Arch Pediatr Adolesc Med*. 2009;163(2):131–40. Review

Sanders LM, Shaw JS, Guez G, Baur C, Rudd R. Health literacy and child health promotion: implications for research, clinical care, and public policy. *Pediatrics*. 2009;124(suppl 3):S306–314

Sanders LM, Zacur G, Haecker T, Klass P. Number of children's books in the home: an indicator of parent health literacy. *Ambul Pediatr*. 2004;4(5):424–428

Schillinger D, Bindman A, Wang F, Stewart A, Piette J. Functional health literacy and the quality of physician-patient communication among diabetes patients. *Patient Educ Couns*. 2004;52(3):315–323

Scott TL, Gazmararian JA, Williams MV, Baker DW. Health literacy and preventive health care use among Medicare enrollees in a managed care organization. *Med Care*. 2002;40(5):395–404

Turner T, Cull WL, Bayldon B, et al. Pediatricians and health literacy: descriptive results from a national survey. *Pediatrics*. 2009;124(sppl 3):S299–S305

Wolf MS, Wilson EA, Rapp DN, et al. Literacy and learning in health care. *Pediatrics*. 2009;124:S275–S281

Yin HS, Mendelsohn AL, Wolf MS, et al. Parents' medication administration errors: role of dosing instruments and health literacy. *Arch Pediatr Adolesc Med*. 2010;164(2):181–186

Yin HS, Dreyer BP, van Schaick L, Foltin GL, Dinglas C, Mendelsohn AL. Randomized controlled trial of a pictogram-based intervention to reduce liquid medication dosing errors and improve adherence among caregivers of young children. *Arch Pediatr Adolesc Med*. 2008;162(9):814–822

Yin HS, Forbis SG, Dreyer BP. Health literacy and pediatric health. *Curr Probl Pediatr Adolesc Health Care*. 2007;37(7):258–286

Screening Tests

REALM

Davis TC, Long SW, Jackson RH, et al. Rapid estimate of adult literacy in medicine: a shortened screening instrument. *Fam Med*. 1993;25:391–395

Bass PF, Wilson JF, Griffith CH, Barnett DR. Residents' ability to identify patients with poor literacy skills. *Acad Med*. 2002;77(10):1039–1041

Health Literacy Measurement Tools. Rockville, MD: Agency for Healthcare Research and Quality; 2009. http://www.ahrq.gov/populations/sahlsatool.htm

S-TOFHLA

Parker RM, Baker DW, Williams MV, Nurss JR. The Test of Functional Health Literacy in Adults: a new instrument for measuring patients' literacy skills. *J Gen Intern Med*. 1995;10:537–541

Baker DW, Williams MV, Parker RM, Gazmararian JA, Nurss J. Development of a brief test to measure functional health literacy. *Patient Educ Couns*. 1999;38(1):33–42

NVS

Weiss BD, Mays MZ, Martz W, et al. Quick assessment of literacy in primary care: the newest vital sign. *Ann Fam Med*. 2005;3:514–22

Other Screening

Chew LD, Bradley KA, Boyko EJ. Brief questions to identify patients with inadequate health literacy. *Fam Med*. 2004;36(8):588–594

Kumar D, Sanders L, Lokker N, et al. *Validation of a New Measure of Parent Health Literacy: The Parent Health Activities Test (PHAT)*. Toronto, Ontario, Canada: Pediatric Academic Societies; 2007

JOSEPH DIFRANZA, MD
ROBERT WELLMAN, PhD

TOBACCO DEPENDENCE

The Hooked on Nicotine Checklist (HONC) is a rapid screening tool for identifying tobacco users who could benefit from assistance with cessation. It identifies when a person has become hooked on tobacco, and can be used with anyone using tobacco. The HONC can be used to help patients realize they are hooked. This may motivate them to quit before it becomes more difficult to do so.

Why Is It Important to Include Tobacco Dependence in History, Observation, and Surveillance?

Adolescents are uniquely susceptible to nicotine. They develop symptoms of dependence very quickly, and they have difficulty quitting smoking. Symptoms of dependence can appear within days of the onset of use, when youths are smoking as little as one cigarette per week. Many youths are hooked before they even think of themselves as smokers.

The age at which youths begin to use tobacco is crucial. Dependence is more severe when use begins during childhood or early adolescence.

Traditional measures of nicotine dependence were developed for adult smokers. They are not sensitive enough to detect the first symptoms of dependence in youths.

Consensus screening recommendations exist. The Public Health Service clinical guideline, *Treating Tobacco Use and Dependence: 2008 Update,* which is endorsed by the American Academy of Pediatrics, provides consensus recommendations to screen pediatric and adolescent patients for tobacco use.

A tobacco screening tool has been developed specifically for use with adolescents. Nicotine dependence can be identified as soon as a smoker has developed any symptom that presents a barrier to

quitting. When quitting requires an effort, the smoker has lost some degree of autonomy over his or her tobacco use. The loss of autonomy is the central feature of dependence.

The HONC is the first measure developed specifically to identify nicotine dependence in youths by measuring their loss of autonomy over tobacco use.

The HONC has strong psychometric properties as evaluated in multiple studies of youths and adults. In a 30-month prospective study of the natural history of tobacco use in a cohort of 679 seventh-grade students, youths who answered yes to one or more items on the HONC were 44 times more likely to be smoking at the end of the study than were smokers who had no positive responses.[1]

The effectiveness of the HONC, or any other tobacco dependence screening tools, in clinical practice has not yet been formally evaluated, although anecdotal reports support its usefulness for screening in clinical settings.

How Should You Screen for Tobacco Dependence?

Administer the HONC either through an interview during an office visit or as part of a self-administered health history form. For users of smokeless tobacco, substitute the word "chew" for "smoke" as appropriate.

The Hooked on Nicotine Checklist

	Yes	No
1. Have you ever tried to quit smoking, but couldn't?		
2. Do you smoke now because it is really hard to quit?		
3. Have you ever felt like you were addicted to tobacco?		
4. Do you ever have strong cravings to smoke?		
5. Have you ever felt like you really needed a cigarette?		
6. Is it hard to keep from smoking in places where you are not supposed to, like school?		
7. When you tried to stop smoking… (or, when you haven't used tobacco for a while…)		
a. Did you find it hard to concentrate because you couldn't smoke?		
b. Did you feel more irritable because you couldn't smoke?		
c. Did you feel a strong need or urge to smoke?		
d. Did you feel nervous, restless, or anxious because you couldn't smoke?		

How Should You Score and Interpret the HONC?

Scoring the HONC

Score the HONC by counting the number of "yes" responses. The number of symptoms a patient endorses, or says yes to, serves as a measure of the extent to which autonomy has been lost. The average HONC score for adolescents who do not smoke every day is 4, while that for adult daily smokers is 7. It is important to note that a score that is below average for the patient's age group is NOT an indication that the patient is not dependent.

Patients who score a zero on the HONC by answering "no" to all 10 questions enjoy full autonomy over their use of tobacco. Because each of the 10 symptoms measured by the HONC has face validity as an indicator of diminished autonomy, patients can be informed that they are hooked if they endorse any symptom.

Interpreting HONC Results

An autonomous smoker can quit without effort or discomfort, just as it takes no effort to stop eating spinach for a day. Autonomy is diminished when there is an obstacle to overcome or a price to be paid for quitting. Each question on the HONC addresses some aspect of diminished autonomy over tobacco.

1. *Have you ever tried to quit smoking but couldn't?*

   A failed cessation attempt is an obvious indication of diminished autonomy. If quitting was effortless, the patient would no longer be smoking.

2. *Do you smoke now because it is really hard to quit?*

   This item is included to capture those who do not want to smoke but have not made an "official" effort to quit, often out of a fear of failure. Because they are doing something they don't want to do, they have diminished autonomy.

3. *Have you ever felt like you were addicted to tobacco?*

   A person with full autonomy over his or her tobacco use would not feel addicted.

4. *Do you ever have strong cravings to smoke?*

   Strong cravings, a symptom of addiction, make quitting difficult and unpleasant.

5. *Have you ever felt like you really needed a cigarette?*

   Smokers feel they really need a cigarette because of cravings, withdrawal symptoms, or psychological dependence. Whatever the reason, quitting is more difficult and autonomy is diminished.

6. *Is it hard to keep from smoking in places where you are not supposed to, like school?*

   An autonomous smoker would have no difficulty refraining from smoking, especially where it is forbidden.

7. *When you tried to stop smoking… OR When you haven't used tobacco for a while…*

   a. *Did you find it hard to concentrate because you couldn't smoke?*

   b. *Did you feel more irritable because you couldn't smoke?*

   c. *Did you feel a strong need or urge to smoke?*

   d. *Did you feel nervous, restless, or anxious because you couldn't smoke?*

All of these questions get at withdrawal symptoms, which make quitting unpleasant and more difficult. A person experiencing these symptoms has diminished autonomy.

What Results Should You Document?

Record the patient's total HONC score. Note any symptoms endorsed, as these should be addressed during cessation counseling.

CPT and *ICD-9-CM* Codes	
305.1	Tobacco use disorder/tobacco dependence
99406	Smoking and tobacco use cessation counseling visit; intermediate, >3 minutes up to 10 minutes.
99407	Intensive, >10 minutes

The American Academy of Pediatrics publishes a complete line of coding publications, including an annual edition of *Coding for Pediatrics*. For more information on these excellent resources, visit the American Academy of Pediatrics Online Bookstore at **www.aap.org/bookstore/**.

These behavior change intervention codes are reported when the service is provided by a physician or other qualified health care professional. The service involves specific validated interventions, including assessing readiness for change and barriers to change, advising change in behavior, providing specific suggested actions and motivational counseling, and arranging for services and follow-up care. The medical record documentation must support the total time spent in performing the service, which may be reported in addition to other separate and distinct services on the same day.

Resources

Articles

American Academy of Pediatrics Committee on Substance Abuse. Tobacco's toll: implications for the pediatrician. *Pediatrics.* 2001;107:794–798

DiFranza JR, Savageau JA, Fletcher K, et al. Measuring the loss of autonomy over nicotine use in adolescents: the DANDY (Development and Assessment of Nicotine Dependence in Youths) Study. *Arch Pediatr Adolesc Med.* 2002;156:397–403

Fiore MC, Bailey WC, Cohen SJ, et al. *Treating Tobacco Use and Dependence: 2008 Update.* Rockville, MD: US Department of Health and Human Services, Public Health Service; 2008

O'Loughlin J, DiFranza J, Tarasuk J, et al. Assessment of nicotine dependence symptoms in adolescents: a comparison of five indicators. *Tob Control.* 2002;11:354–360

Wellman RJ, DiFranza JR, Pbert L, et al. A comparison of the psychometric properties of the Hooked on Nicotine Checklist and the Modified Fagerström Tolerance Questionnaire. *Addict Behav.* 2006;31:486–495

Wheeler KC, Fletcher KE, Wellman RJ, DiFranza JR. Screening adolescents for nicotine dependence: the Hooked on Nicotine Checklist. *J Adolesc Health.* 2004;35:225–230

Screening Instruments

The HONC is available at http://whyquit.com/whyquit/LinksYouth.html. It is available in several languages.

Reference

1. DiFranza JR, Savageau JA, Rigotti NA, et al. The development of symptoms of tobacco dependence in youths: 30-month follow-up data from the DANDY study. *Tob Control.* 2002;11:228–235

PHYSICAL EXAMINATION

A complete physical examination is included as part of every Bright Futures visit. The examination must be comprehensive and also focus on specific assessments that are appropriate for the child's or adolescent's age, developmental phase, and needs. This portion of the visit builds on the history gathered earlier. The physical examination also provides opportunities to identify silent or subtle illnesses or conditions and time for the health care professional to educate children and their parents about the body and its growth and development.

The chapters in this section of the book focus on topics that emerge during the examination. **Assessing Growth and Nutrition; Sexual Maturity Stages; In-toeing and Out-toeing;** and **Spine, Hip, and Knee** discuss critical aspects of healthy development that must be assessed with regularity. **Blood Pressure and Early Childhood Caries** examine issues of vital public health importance and provide updated guidelines. **Sports Participation** provides useful guidance for health care professionals at a time when increased physical activity among children and adolescents is a priority.

SUSANNE TANSKI, MD, MPH
LYNN C. GARFUNKEL, MD

ASSESSING GROWTH AND NUTRITION

Accurate and reliable physical measures are used to monitor the growth of an individual, detect growth abnormalities, monitor nutritional status, and track the effects of medical or nutritional intervention. As such, they are essential components of the physical examination. This chapter reviews measurement of length, height, weight, and head circumference and calculation of body mass index (BMI).

PHYSICAL EXAMINATION

Why Is It Important to Assess Growth and Nutrition During the Physical Examination?

Growth measurements correlate directly to nutritional status and can indicate whether a child's health and well-being are at risk.[1] Deviations from normal growth patterns may be familial patterns but may indicate medical problems.[2] For example, abnormal linear growth or poor weight gain could indicate a variety of medical problems, including malnutrition, chronic illness, psychosocial deprivation, hormonal disorders, or syndromes with dwarfism.[3] Similarly, growth trajectories that deviate above the norm (increased weight for height [or increased BMI]) can also indicate medical problems with adverse consequences. Monitoring growth and deviations from normal patterns can help detect and allow intervention for many medical conditions and abnormalities.[2]

Calculating and tracking BMI provides vital information about weight status and risk of overweight and obesity. Body mass index is a clinically useful weight-for-height index that reflects excess body fat as well as nutritional status.[4,5]

Obesity in childhood is associated with immediate and long-term adverse health and psychosocial outcomes, leading to health problems in as many as 50% of US children.[2] Obesity in children has been associated with increased blood pressure, total cholesterol, low-density lipoprotein cholesterol, and triglycerides and low levels of high-density lipoprotein cholesterol.[5]

The American Academy of Pediatrics and American Academy of Family Physicians endorse universal screening of BMI and use of BMI growth curves for plotting BMI percentiles to identify obese and overweight children.

Measuring head circumference, especially within the first 3 years, may identify neurologic abnormalities as well as malnutrition.[5,6] Identification of abnormal growth patterns can lead to early diagnosis of treatable conditions, such as hydrocephalous, or identification of disorders associated with slowed head growth, such as Rett syndrome.[7]

How Should You Take These Measurements?

General Considerations

The measurement process has 2 steps—measure and record. Accurate weighing and measuring have 3 critical components—technique, equipment, and trained measurers. You must use the appropriate techniques for each measurement.

Your choice of whether to use English or metric units for measurements and plotting can depend on a variety of circumstances. If the available equipment is accurately calibrated and the measurers follow standard procedures, then you can record data in either English or metric units. The use of metric measures is encouraged when weighing infants, children, and adolescents in a clinical setting. To convert from kilograms to pounds, multiply the kilogram amount by 2.2 (eg, 50 kg x 2.2 = 110 lb).

Consistent procedures must be used. If measures are in error, then the foundation of the growth assessment is also in error. It is important to record the date, age, and actual measurements so the data can be used by others or at a later time.

Measure Stature (Length or Height)

Infancy and Early Childhood (0–2 years)

- Until they can stand securely (age 2 years), measure infants lying down in a supine position on a measuring frame or an examining table.

- Align the infant's head snugly against the top bar of the frame and ask an assistant to secure it there. Parents can help restrain infants for length measurements, as it is a painless procedure.

- Straighten the infant's body, hips, and knees.

- Hold the infant's feet in a vertical position (long axis of foot perpendicular to long axis of leg). Bring the foot board snugly against the bottom of the foot. Some authorities suggest measuring twice and taking an average.

- If an examining table is used, mark the spots at the top of the child's head and bottom of feet and then measure between the marks. (Note that this is not ideal as it is difficult to get an accurate length using this technique.)

- Plot length measurements on a standard growth chart for age and gender, or one appropriate for the child (eg, low birth weight infant, infant with trisomy 21, infant with Turner syndrome).

Child (2 years and older)

- Have the child remove his or her shoes.

- Have the child stand up with the bottom of the heels on floor and back of foot touching the wall, knees straight, scapula and occiput also on the wall, looking straight ahead with head held level.

- Align the measuring bar perpendicular to the wall and parallel to the floor (on a stadiometer or other measuring rod) with the top of the head.

- If a scale with a measuring bar is not available, place a flat object such as a clipboard on the child's head in a horizontal position and read the height at the point at which the object touches a measuring tape on the back of the scale or a flat wall surface.

- Plot height measurements on a standardized growth chart for age and gender, or one appropriate for the child.

Measure Weight

Infancy and Early Childhood

- Weigh younger infants nude or in a clean diaper on a calibrated beam or electronic scale. Weigh older infants in a clean, disposable diaper.

- Position the infant in the center of the scale tray.

- It is desirable for 2 people to be involved when weighing an infant. One measurer weighs the infant and protects him or her from harm (such as falling) and reads the weight as it is obtained. The other measurer immediately notes the measurement in the infant's chart.

- Weigh the infant to the nearest 0.01 kg or 1/2 oz.

- Record the weight as soon as it is completed.

- Then reposition the infant and repeat the weight measurement. Note the second measurement in writing. Compare the weights. They should agree within 0.1 kg or 1/4 lb. If the difference exceeds this, reweigh the infant a third time. Record the average of the 2 closest weights.

If an infant is too active or too distressed for an accurate weight measurement, try the following options:

- Postpone the measurement until later in the visit when the infant may be more comfortable with the setting.

- If you have an electronic scale, use this alternative measurement technique: Have the parent stand on the scale and reset the scale to zero. Then have the parent hold the infant and read the infant's weight.

Child

- A child older than 36 months who can stand without assistance should be weighed standing on a scale using a calibrated beam balance or electronic scale.

- Have the child or adolescent wear only lightweight undergarments or a gown.

- Have the child or adolescent stand on the center of the platform of the scale.

- Record the weight of the individual to the nearest 0.01 kg or 1/2 oz. (If the scale is not digital, record to the nearest half-kilo or pound). Record the weight on the chart.

- Reposition the individual and repeat the weight measure.

- Compare the measures. They should agree within 0.1 kg or 1/4 lb. (If the scale is not digital, compare to the nearest half-kilo or pound.) If the difference between the measures exceeds the tolerance limit, reposition the child and measure a third time. Record the average of the 2 measures in closest agreement.

In the standardized scale for children, all weights between the 5th and 85th percentiles are considered normal. As important as the fact that a child's weight falls between these percentiles on a growth chart is that over time the weight follows one of the percentile curves. In other words, a child who is at the 80th percentile the first time he or she is weighed and at the 40th percentile a month later is cause for concern. A child is defined as having a failure to thrive syndrome (a medical diagnosis) if height or weight drops below the third percentile on a standardized growth chart.

Calculate BMI

- Choose English or metric calculation for BMI.

  ▷ English: (Weight (lb) / [Stature (in) x Stature (in)]) x 703

  ▷ Metric: Weight (kg) / [Stature (m) x Stature (m)]

- Plot the child's or adolescent's BMI on a growth chart for age and sex to determine BMI percentile. In the United States, BMI growth charts are available for ages 2 to 20. Alternatively, the Centers for Disease Control and Prevention (CDC) has a Web-based tool to calculate both the BMI and age- and sex-adjusted BMI percentile (http://apps.nccd.cdc.gov/dnpabmi/Calculator.aspx). See the Resources section for further details.

Measure Head Circumference

Obtain an accurate head circumference, or occipital frontal circumference, by using a flexible non-stretchable measuring tape. Head circumference is generally measured on infants and children until the age of 3 years.

Measure head circumference over the largest circumference of the head, namely the most prominent part on the back of the head (occiput) and just above the eyebrows (supraorbital ridges).

- Place a tape measure around an infant's head just above the eyebrows and around the most prominent portion of the back of the head, the occipital prominence.

- Pull the tape snugly to compress the hair and underlying soft tissues. Read the measurement to the nearest 0.1 cm or 1/8 inch and record on the chart.

- Reposition the tape and remeasure the head circumference. The measures should agree within 0.2 cm or 1/4 inch. If the difference between the measures exceeds the tolerance limit, the infant should be repositioned and remeasured a third time. The average of the 2 measures in closest agreement is recorded.

- Plot measurements on a standardized growth chart for age and gender.

- Head circumference should correlate with the child's length (eg, if length is in the 40th percentile, head circumference should also be 40th percentile).

What Should You Do With an Abnormal Result?

Stature

- Children who fall off their height curves (decline in stature/length percentiles or present with extreme short stature) may need to undergo evaluations for underlying medical problems.

- First, be sure that the measurements are accurate, make sense, and are appropriately plotted.

- Calculate mean parental height and plot.

  ▸ Mean parental height calculation: Add parental heights and subtract 5 inches for a girl (from Dad's height) or add 5 inches (to Mom's height) for a boy, and then divide that entire number by 2.

  Example: mother is 5'4" (64"), father is 5'9" (69"): (5'9" + 5'4") +/- 5")/2 = mean parental height. A girl's mean parental height would be 5'4" and a boy's would be 5'9 ". (These are average heights for male and female population.)

  ▸ If the child is short, but mean parental height falls in the same percentile, the child may have familial short stature.

  ▸ If the parents entered puberty late and the child is short and prepubertal at a time when most children are in puberty, he or she may have constitutional delay.

  ▸ These children all need to be followed closely and evaluated or referred to an appropriate specialist.

- Those with short stature may need to be assessed for endocrinopathies, pubertal delay, boney dysplasias, or syndromes. Pubertal delays may be genetic/familial or be due to an underlying medical condition

Weight/BMI

- Drop in weight percentiles by more than one large percentile or presentation with extreme underweight may warrant further investigation.

- First be sure measurements are correct and were plotted correctly.

- A number of medical conditions can present with weight loss or fall off weight growth curves, including malabsorption, renal disease, cardiac disorders, neurologic and pulmonary disorders, food or feeding abnormalities, family or environmental difficulties, and chronic infections. Workup and potential referral should proceed as suggested by history and physical examination.

- Review the "Weight Maintenance and Weight Loss" and "Metabolic Syndrome" chapters in this volume for issues with overweight/obesity.

Head Circumference

Consider the following actions for a child with an abnormal head size:

- Accurately measure the head circumference and assess the pattern of head growth. If previous measurements are available, assess the onset of the abnormal head size.

- Inspect and palpate the skull.

- Compare the head circumference with other growth parameters.

- Observe for the presence or absence of dysmorphic features.

- Note the presence or absence of congenital abnormalities involving other organ systems.

- Measure the head sizes of first-degree relatives.

- Conduct neurologic and developmental assessments that may

  ▸ Reveal asymmetries

  ▸ Abnormalities in muscle tone, posture, strength, and reflexes

  ▸ Generalized psychomotor retardation

  ▸ Motor delays

  ▸ Speech or language and cognitive impairments

  ▸ Autistic features

- Assess for signs and symptoms of increased intracranial pressure.

What Results Should You Document?

Plot height, weight, and BMI measurements in the child's growth charts. It is essential to select the appropriate chart for the age and sex of the child or adolescent. The CDC growth charts are presented as

Sex and Age	Charts
Boys, birth to 36 mos	Weight-for-length
Boys, birth to 36 mos	Weight-for-age
Boys, birth to 36 mos	Length-for-age
Boys, birth to 36 mos	Head circumference-for-age
Girls, birth to 36 mos	Weight-for-length
Girls, birth to 36 mos	Weight-for-age
Girls, birth to 36 mos	Length-for-age
Girls, birth to 36 mos	Head circumference-for-age
Boys, 2 to 20 yrs	BMI-for-age
Boys, 2 to 20 yrs	Weight-for-age
Boys, 2 to 20 yrs	Stature-for-age
Girls, 2 to 20 yrs	BMI-for-age
Girls, 2 to 20 yrs	Weight-for-age
Girls, 2 to 20 yrs	Stature-for-age
Boys 2 to 5 yrs	Weight-for-stature (optional)
Girls 2 to 5 yrs	Weight-for-stature (optional)

For children between ages 2 and 3, the measurement you obtain must match the graph you use (eg, if supine length is measured, use the 0–3 years length-for-age graph, not the 2–20 stature [standing height]-for-age graph).

A straight edge, right angle triangle or commercially available plotting aid is recommended to locate the intersecting point of the axis values. After graphing a set of measurements, check to see if they are consistent with those from previous visits (ie, the child is on roughly the same percentile lines as before). If not, check the measurements, graphing, or both.

When you have made accurate measurements, calculated age correctly, and plotted them on the appropriate growth chart, use the information in the clinical assessment process. Share the information with the family (ie, translate the measurements into a form that is useful to them).

ICD-9-CM Codes

259.4	Dwarfism
253.0	Gigantism (cerebral, hypophyseal, pituitary)
331.4	Hydrocephalus (acquired, external, internal, malignant, noncommunicating, obstructive, recurrent)
756.0	Macrocephaly
742.4	Megalencephaly
742.1	Microcephaly
278.00	Obesity (constitutional, exogenous, familial, nutritional, simple)*
278.01	Obesity, morbid*
278.01	Obesity, severe*
278.00	Overweight*
783.2	Abnormal loss of weight and underweight (use BMI code if known, V85.0)
783.21	Loss of weight
783.22	Underweight
783.41	Failure to thrive, poor weight gain
783.43	Short stature
783.3	Feeding problem
779.3	Newborn feeding problem

*Obesity codes are not reimbursed in all jurisdictions. Practitioners may select additional diagnoses.

The American Academy of Pediatrics publishes a complete line of coding publications, including an annual edition of *Coding for Pediatrics*. For more information on these excellent resources, visit the American Academy of Pediatrics Online Bookstore at **www.aap.org/bookstore/**.

Resources

Articles

Childhood Obesity Working Group, US Preventive Task Force. Screening for overweight in children and adolescents: where is the evidence? A commentary by the Childhood Obesity Working Group of the US Preventive Services Task Force. *Pediatrics*. 2005;116(1):235–238

Centers for Disease Control and Prevention. *Identification and Quantification of Sources of Error in Weighing and Measuring Children.* Atlanta, GA: Centers for Disease Control and Prevention, Public Health Service, and US Department of Health, Education, and Welfare; 1976

Lohman TG, Roche AF, Martorell R. *Anthropometric Standardization Reference Manual.* Champaign, IL: Human Kinetics Books; 1988

Mei Z, Grummer-Strawn LM, Pietrobelli A, Goulding A, Goran MI, Dietz WH. Validity of body mass index compared with other body-composition screening indexes for the assessment of body fatness in children and adolescents. *Am J Clin Nutr.* 2002;75:978–985

Pillitteri A. *Maternal and Child Health Nursing: Care of the Childbearing and Childrearing Family.* 5th ed. Philadelphia, PA: Lippincott Williams and Wilkins; 2007

Third National Health and Nutrition Examination (NHANES III) Anthropometric Procedures Video. National Center for Health Statistics Web Site. 2008. http://www.cdc.gov/nchs/products/elec_prods/subject/video.htm

Scales or Tools

Centers for Disease Control and Prevention: BMI Percent Calculator for Child and Teen: http://apps.nccd.cdc.gov/dnpabmi/Calculator.aspx

National Center for Health Statistics: Clinical Growth Charts: http://www.cdc.gov/growthcharts/

References

1. Barness LA. Section 1: Introduction to Pediatrics, Chapter 5: Pediatric history and physical examination. In: McMillan JA, Feigin RD, DeAngelis CD, Jones MD, eds. *Oski's Pediatrics: Principles and Practice.* 4th ed. Philadelphia, PA: Lippincott Williams and Wilkins; 2006:33

2. Purugganan OH. In brief: abnormalities in head size. *Pediatr Rev.* 2006;27:473–476

3. Centers for Disease Control and Prevention and Health Service Administration. *Weighing and Measuring Children: A Training Manual for Supervisory Personnel.* Atlanta, GA: Centers for Disease Control and Prevention; 1980

4. Barlow SE, Dietz WH. Obesity evaluation and treatment: expert committee recommendations. *Pediatrics.* 1998;102(3):e29

5. Beker L. In brief: principles of growth assessment. *Pediatr Rev.* 2006;27:196–198

6. Sulkes SB. Section II: Growth and development. In: Nelson WE, Behrman RE, Kliegman RM, eds. *Nelson Essentials of Pediatrics.* 3rd ed. Philadelphia, PA: W.B. Saunders Co; 1998:1

7. Nellhaus G. Head circumference from birth to eighteen years: practical composite international and interracial graphs. *Pediatrics.* 1968;41:106–114

MARC LANDE, MD
WILLIAM VARADE, MD

BLOOD PRESSURE

The following guidelines are adapted directly from the "Fourth Report on the Diagnosis, Evaluation, and Treatment of High Blood Pressure in Children and Adolescents."[1]

Why Is It Important to Assess Blood Pressure During the Physical Examination?

High blood pressure is a growing health concern for children and adolescents. A large national database shows that the prevalence of high blood pressure (BP) in children and adolescents is increasing. These increases are even larger than would be expected from the increase in obesity prevalence.

Primary hypertension is detectable in children and adolescents. Moreover, it is a common problem.

The long-term health risks of hypertension can be substantial. Target-organ damage is commonly associated with hypertension in children and adolescents. Left ventricular hypertrophy, the most prominent finding, is present in up to 36% of hypertensive children.

In addition, elevated BP in childhood correlates with the presence of hypertension in adulthood.

Obesity and hypertension are linked. The prevalence of children who are overweight is increasing. Children and adolescents with hypertension are frequently overweight, with hypertension present in approximately 30% of overweight children. Given the marked increase in childhood obesity, hypertension is becoming a significant health issue.

How Is Hypertension Defined in Children and Adolescents?

Blood pressure falls into several categories.

- **Prehypertension** is systolic BP and/or diastolic BP ≥90th percentile but <95th percentile for age, sex, and height.

  Adolescents with BP ≥120/80 should be considered **prehypertensive,** even if 120/80 is less than the 90th percentile.

- **White-coat hypertension** is BP at ≥95th percentile in the office, normal outside of the office setting. Ambulatory BP monitoring is often needed to make this diagnosis.

- **Hypertension** is defined as systolic BP and/or diastolic BP ≥95th percentile for age, sex, and height on 3 or more occasions. Hypertensive children are further categorized into 2 stages.

  - Stage 1: BP ≥95th percentile but <5 mm Hg above the 99th percentile (<99th percentile + 5 mm Hg)

  - Stage 2: BP is >5 mm Hg above the 99th percentile (>99th percentile + 5 mm Hg)

See the Resources section of this chapter for National Heart, Lung, and Blood Institute blood pressure tables for children and adolescents.

When and How Should You Measure Blood Pressure?

When to Measure

- Children younger than 3 years should have their BP measured under the following circumstances:

  ▶ History of prematurity, low birth weight, care in the neonatal intensive care unit

  ▶ Congenital heart disease

  ▶ Renal or urologic disease

  ▶ Family history of congenital renal disease

  ▶ Solid-organ or bone marrow transplant

  ▶ History of malignancy

  ▶ Treatment with drugs known to raise BP

  ▶ Any systemic illness associated with hypertension

  ▶ Elevated intracranial pressure

- Children older than 3 years should have their BP routinely measured.

How to Measure

- Position the child.

  ▶ Child should be sitting quietly for 5 minutes prior to taking BP

  ▶ Back supported with feet on floor

  ▶ Right arm supported with cubital fossa at heart level

- Use the appropriate cuff size.

  ▶ Inflatable bladder width should be at least 40% of the arm circumference at the midpoint between the olecranon and acromion.

  ▶ Cuff bladder length should cover 80% to 100% of the arm circumference.

  ▶ If a cuff is too small, use the next largest cuff, even if it appears too large.

- Take the measurement.

  ▶ If possible, use the right arm. This will make the measurement consistent with national norms and will prevent confusion with the effects of potential coarctation.

  ▶ Place stethoscope over brachial artery pulse, proximal and medial to the cubital fossa, below the bottom edge of the cuff.

  ▶ Consider using the bell of the stethoscope; it may allow softer Korotkoff sounds to be heard.

  ▶ Determine the systolic BP by the onset of Korotkoff sounds (K1).

  ▶ Determine the diastolic BP by the disappearance of Korotkoff sounds (K5).

  ▶ In some children, Korotkoff sounds can be heard all the way to 0. In this situation, repeat the BP with less pressure on the stethoscope head.

  ▶ If Korotkoff sounds still go to 0, then record muffling of the Korotkoff sounds (K4) as the diastolic BP.

What Should You Do With an Abnormal Result?

Children and adolescents with persistent prehypertension (>6 months in duration) who are overweight, have diabetes, kidney disease, or Stage 1 hypertension should have the appropriate evaluation for secondary hypertension and target-organ damage as recommended in the "Fourth Report on the Diagnosis, Evaluation, and Treatment of High Blood Pressure in Children and Adolescents."[1]

Children and adolescents with persistent Stage 1 hypertension, despite a trial of lifestyle modification, may need antihypertensive medications. Consider referral to a practitioner with expertise in pediatric hypertension.

Consider early referral to a practitioner with expertise in pediatric hypertension for all children and adolescents with Stage 2 hypertension.

What Results Should You Document?

Document routine blood pressures in the medical record with other vital signs. Record prehypertension and stage of hypertension in the problem list.

ICD-9-CM Codes	
796.2	Elevation of blood pressure, no diagnosis of hypertension
401.1	Hypertension, benign
401.0	Hypertension, malignant

The American Academy of Pediatrics publishes a complete line of coding publications including an annual edition of *Coding for Pediatrics*. For more information on these excellent resources, visit the American Academy of Pediatrics online bookstore at **www.aap.org/bookstore/.**

Resources

Tools

National Heart, Lung, and Blood Institute

Blood Pressure Tables for Children and Adolescents: http://www.nhlbi.nih.gov/guidelines/hypertension/child_tbl.htm

Article

Muntner P, He J, Cutler JA, Wildman RP, Whelton PK. Trends in blood pressure among children and adolescents. *JAMA.* 2004;291:2107–2113

Web Sites

American Heart Association: http://www.heart.org/HEARTORG/

High Blood Pressure in Children: http://www.americanheart.org/presenter.jhtml?identifier=4609

International Pediatric Hypertension Association: http://www.pediatrichypertension.org

Reference

1   National High Blood Pressure Education Program Working Group on High Blood Pressure in Children and Adolescents. The fourth report on the diagnosis, evaluation, and treatment of high blood pressure in children and adolescents. *Pediatrics.* 2004;114:555–576

PHYSICAL EXAMINATION

Blood Pressure Levels for Boys by Age and Height Percentile

Age (Year)	BP Percentile ↓	Systolic BP (mmHg) ← Percentile of Height →							Diastolic BP (mmHg) ← Percentile of Height →						
		5th	10th	25th	50th	75th	90th	95th	5th	10th	25th	50th	75th	90th	95th
1	50th	80	81	83	85	87	88	89	34	35	36	37	38	39	39
	90th	94	95	97	99	100	102	103	49	50	51	52	53	53	54
	95th	98	99	101	103	104	106	106	54	54	55	56	57	58	58
	99th	105	106	108	110	112	113	114	61	62	63	64	65	66	66
2	50th	84	85	87	88	90	92	92	39	40	41	42	43	44	44
	90th	97	99	100	102	104	105	106	54	55	56	57	58	58	59
	95th	101	102	104	106	108	109	110	59	59	60	61	62	63	63
	99th	109	110	111	113	115	117	117	66	67	68	69	70	71	71
3	50th	86	87	89	91	93	94	95	44	44	45	46	47	48	48
	90th	100	101	103	105	107	108	109	59	59	60	61	62	63	63
	95th	104	105	107	109	110	112	113	63	63	64	65	66	67	67
	99th	111	112	114	116	118	119	120	71	71	72	73	74	75	75
4	50th	88	89	91	93	95	96	97	47	48	49	50	51	51	52
	90th	102	103	105	107	109	110	111	62	63	64	65	66	66	67
	95th	106	107	109	111	112	114	115	66	67	68	69	70	71	71
	99th	113	114	116	118	120	121	122	74	75	76	77	78	78	79
5	50th	90	91	93	95	96	98	98	50	51	52	53	54	55	55
	90th	104	105	106	108	110	111	112	65	66	67	68	69	69	70
	95th	108	109	110	112	114	115	116	69	70	71	72	73	74	74
	99th	115	116	118	120	121	123	123	77	78	79	80	81	81	82
6	50th	91	92	94	96	98	99	100	53	53	54	55	56	57	57
	90th	105	106	108	110	111	113	113	68	68	69	70	71	72	72
	95th	109	110	112	114	115	117	117	72	72	73	74	75	76	76
	99th	116	117	119	121	123	124	125	80	80	81	82	83	84	84
7	50th	92	94	95	97	99	100	101	55	55	56	57	58	59	59
	90th	106	107	109	111	113	114	115	70	70	71	72	73	74	74
	95th	110	111	113	115	117	118	119	74	74	75	76	77	78	78
	99th	117	118	120	122	124	125	126	82	82	83	84	85	86	86
8	50th	94	95	97	99	100	102	102	56	57	58	59	60	60	61
	90th	107	109	110	112	114	115	116	71	72	72	73	74	75	76
	95th	111	112	114	116	118	119	120	75	76	77	78	79	79	80
	99th	119	120	122	123	125	127	127	83	84	85	86	87	87	88
9	50th	95	96	98	100	102	103	104	57	58	59	60	61	61	62
	90th	109	110	112	114	115	117	118	72	73	74	75	76	76	77
	95th	113	114	116	118	119	121	121	76	77	78	79	80	81	81
	99th	120	121	123	125	127	128	129	84	85	86	87	88	88	89
10	50th	97	98	100	102	103	105	106	58	59	60	61	61	62	63
	90th	111	112	114	115	117	119	119	73	73	74	75	76	77	78
	95th	115	116	117	119	121	122	123	77	78	79	80	81	81	82
	99th	122	123	125	127	128	130	130	85	86	86	88	88	89	90

Blood Pressure Levels for Boys by Age and Height Percentile (Continued)

Age (Year)	BP Percentile ↓	Systolic BP (mmHg)							Diastolic BP (mmHg)						
		← Percentile of Height →							← Percentile of Height →						
		5th	10th	25th	50th	75th	90th	95th	5th	10th	25th	50th	75th	90th	95th
11	50th	99	100	102	104	105	107	107	59	59	60	61	62	63	63
	90th	113	114	115	117	119	120	121	74	74	75	76	77	78	78
	95th	117	118	119	121	123	124	125	78	78	79	80	81	82	82
	99th	124	125	127	129	130	132	132	86	86	87	88	89	90	90
12	50th	101	102	104	106	108	109	110	59	60	61	62	63	63	64
	90th	115	116	118	120	121	123	123	74	75	75	76	77	78	79
	95th	119	120	122	123	125	127	127	78	79	80	81	82	82	83
	99th	126	127	129	131	133	134	135	86	87	88	89	90	90	91
13	50th	104	105	106	108	110	111	112	60	60	61	62	63	64	64
	90th	117	118	120	122	124	125	126	75	75	76	77	78	79	79
	95th	121	122	124	126	128	129	130	79	79	80	81	82	83	83
	99th	128	130	131	133	135	136	137	87	87	88	89	90	91	91
14	50th	106	107	109	111	113	114	115	60	61	62	63	64	65	65
	90th	120	121	123	125	126	128	128	75	76	77	78	79	79	80
	95th	124	125	127	128	130	132	132	80	80	81	82	83	84	84
	99th	131	132	134	136	138	139	140	87	88	89	90	91	92	92
15	50th	109	110	112	113	115	117	117	61	62	63	64	65	66	66
	90th	122	124	125	127	129	130	131	76	77	78	79	80	80	81
	95th	126	127	129	131	133	134	135	81	81	82	83	84	85	85
	99th	134	135	136	138	140	142	142	88	89	90	91	92	93	93
16	50th	111	112	114	116	118	119	120	63	63	64	65	66	67	67
	90th	125	126	128	130	131	133	134	78	78	79	80	81	82	82
	95th	129	130	132	134	135	137	137	82	83	83	84	85	86	87
	99th	136	137	139	141	143	144	145	90	90	91	92	93	94	94
17	50th	114	115	116	118	120	121	122	65	66	66	67	68	69	70
	90th	127	128	130	132	134	135	136	80	80	81	82	83	84	84
	95th	131	132	134	136	138	139	140	84	85	86	87	87	88	89
	99th	139	140	141	143	145	146	147	92	93	93	94	95	96	97

BP, blood pressure

* The 90th percentile is 1.28 SD, 95th percentile is 1.645 SD, and the 99th percentile is 2.326 SD over the mean.

For research purposes, the standard deviations in Appendix Table B–1 allow one to compute BP Z-scores and percentiles for boys with height percentiles given in Table 3 (i.e., the 5th,10th, 25th, 50th, 75th, 90th, and 95th percentiles). These height percentiles must be converted to height Z-scores given by (5% = -1.645; 10% = -1.28; 25% = -0.68; 50% = 0; 75% = 0.68; 90% = 1.28%; 95% = 1.645) and then computed according to the methodology in steps 2–4 described in Appendix B. For children with height percentiles other than these, follow steps 1–4 as described in Appendix B.

Blood Pressure Levels for Girls by Age and Height Percentile

Age (Year)	BP Percentile ↓	Systolic BP (mmHg) ← Percentile of Height →							Diastolic BP (mmHg) ← Percentile of Height →						
		5th	10th	25th	50th	75th	90th	95th	5th	10th	25th	50th	75th	90th	95th
1	50th	83	84	85	86	88	89	90	38	39	39	40	41	41	42
	90th	97	97	98	100	101	102	103	52	53	53	54	55	55	56
	95th	100	101	102	104	105	106	107	56	57	57	58	59	59	60
	99th	108	108	109	111	112	113	114	64	64	65	65	66	67	67
2	50th	85	85	87	88	89	91	91	43	44	44	45	46	46	47
	90th	98	99	100	101	103	104	105	57	58	58	59	60	61	61
	95th	102	103	104	105	107	108	109	61	62	62	63	64	65	65
	99th	109	110	111	112	114	115	116	69	69	70	70	71	72	72
3	50th	86	87	88	89	91	92	93	47	48	48	49	50	50	51
	90th	100	100	102	103	104	106	106	61	62	62	63	64	64	65
	95th	104	104	105	107	108	109	110	65	66	66	67	68	68	69
	99th	111	111	113	114	115	116	117	73	73	74	74	75	76	76
4	50th	88	88	90	91	92	94	94	50	50	51	52	52	53	54
	90th	101	102	103	104	106	107	108	64	64	65	66	67	67	68
	95th	105	106	107	108	110	111	112	68	68	69	70	71	71	72
	99th	112	113	114	115	117	118	119	76	76	76	77	78	79	79
5	50th	89	90	91	93	94	95	96	52	53	53	54	55	55	56
	90th	103	103	105	106	107	109	109	66	67	67	68	69	69	70
	95th	107	107	108	110	111	112	113	70	71	71	72	73	73	74
	99th	114	114	116	117	118	120	120	78	78	79	79	80	81	81
6	50th	91	92	93	94	96	97	98	54	54	55	56	56	57	58
	90th	104	105	106	108	109	110	111	68	68	69	70	70	71	72
	95th	108	109	110	111	113	114	115	72	72	73	74	74	75	76
	99th	115	116	117	119	120	121	122	80	80	80	81	82	83	83
7	50th	93	93	95	96	97	99	99	55	56	56	57	58	58	59
	90th	106	107	108	109	111	112	113	69	70	70	71	72	72	73
	95th	110	111	112	113	115	116	116	73	74	74	75	76	76	77
	99th	117	118	119	120	122	123	124	81	81	82	82	83	84	84
8	50th	95	95	96	98	99	100	101	57	57	57	58	59	60	60
	90th	108	109	110	111	113	114	114	71	71	71	72	73	74	74
	95th	112	112	114	115	116	118	118	75	75	75	76	77	78	78
	99th	119	120	121	122	123	125	125	82	82	83	83	84	85	86
9	50th	96	97	98	100	101	102	103	58	58	58	59	60	61	61
	90th	110	110	112	113	114	116	116	72	72	72	73	74	75	75
	95th	114	114	115	117	118	119	120	76	76	76	77	78	79	79
	99th	121	121	123	124	125	127	127	83	83	84	84	85	86	87
10	50th	98	99	100	102	103	104	105	59	59	59	60	61	62	62
	90th	112	112	114	115	116	118	118	73	73	73	74	75	76	76
	95th	116	116	117	119	120	121	122	77	77	77	78	79	80	80
	99th	123	123	125	126	127	129	129	84	84	85	86	86	87	88

Resources

Suppliers of fluoride varnish

Fluoride Name	Manufacturer	Colophonium Resin[a]	Supply Company	Unit Dose	Multiple Doses in 1 Tube	Fluoride
AllSolutions	Dentsply Professional 800/989-8826 www.dentsply.com		Patterson 800/552-1260	0.25 mL		5% NaF
Cavity Shield	Omnii/3M ESPE 800/445-3386	Yes	Patterson, RJM, Darby, Sullivan-Schein, others	0.25 mL 0.40 mL		5% NaF
White Varnish[a]	3M ESPE 800/445-3386	No	Same as above	0.25 mL 0.4 mL 0.4 mL		5% NaF
Durafluor	Medicom 800/361-2862	Yes	Patterson 800/552-1260	0.25 mL 0.4 mL	10-mL tube, brushes separate	5% NaF
Duraphat	Colgate Oral Pharmaceuticals	Yes	Colgate Oral Pharmaceuticals	No	10-mL tube (Purchase brushes separately from Henry Schein: 800/372-4346.)	5% NaF
Fluo-Protector	Ivoclar North America Vivadent 800/327-4688	Polyurathane base	Patterson	0.4 mL		0.1% difluoro-silane
VarnishAmerica	Medical Product Laboratores 800/523-0191	No	Direct sales	0.25 mL 04 mL		5% NaF
Topex DuroShield	Sultan Healthcare 800/238-6739	Yes + xylitol	Patterson or Darby	0.4 mL		5% NaF

[a]White Varnish from 3M ESPE is available without the colophonium resin. Omni claimed that some people are allergic to colophonium and this offers an alternative. It also has a total of 0.5 mL in each unit dose container, and the practitioner would use a dispensing guide to use the desired amount (eg, 0.25, 0.4, or 0.5 mL). Since it is a unit dose intended for one person, the amount not used is wasted. if you have a child that doesn't have a full set of primary teeth.
The listing of brand names does not imply endorsement.

Dental Supply Companies

Darby	800/645-2310
Patterson	800/328-5536
Dental City	800/292-7910
Sullivan Schein	800/372-4326

DONNA PHILLIPS, MD

INTOEING AND OUTTOEING

Given the prevalence of rotational findings of the lower extremities in early childhood, including intoeing, and outtoeing, it is important to understand when additional studies and referral are necessary. While Bright Futures does not have specific recommendations regarding orthopedic assessments during early childhood, the editors determined that these conditions are sufficiently important and common to include in this handbook.

Why Is It Important to Assess Orthopedic Issues During the Physical Examination?

Many children who toe in or toe out are normal. Similarly, an appearance of knock knees and bow legs can be normal. It can be of great concern to parents. Our task is to distinguish normal from abnormal. If normal, knowledge of the etiology and the natural history is reassuring to the parents. If the condition is thought to be abnormal, appropriate studies and referrals can be made.

How Should You Perform These Examinations?

The evaluation of the child needs to begin with a history. Including the following questions:

- What do parents see that they are concerned about?
- When did they first notice the problem?
- Has it changed over time? Is it better? Is it worse? Is it just different?
- What is the family history? Did anyone else have the problem as a child or persisting into adulthood?
- What is the child's birth history?
- Have they reached the appropriate developmental milestones?
- What is the child's diet?

While taking the history, it is useful to observe the undressed child playing in the examination room. It is also imperative that a long hallway is used to observe the child run or walk and observe their gait. The specific examinations for different conditions are as follows.

Intoeing and Outtoeing

Toeing in or out may come from the hip, tibia or foot. Evaluation for each of these includes observing the child walking or running. Estimate the foot progression angle, which is the degrees that the foot points in (a negative foot progression angle) or points out (a positive foot progression angle) relative to a straight line.

To discover where the toeing in or toeing out is coming from you must assess the hip range of motion, assess the tibial torsion, and examine the feet.

Hip Rotation Evaluation

With young or fearful children, examine them on their parent's lap. With the child's hips flexed to a right angle, internally and externally rotate the hips. Lie the child down on the lap and do the same examination with the hips extended. Estimate the degree of internal and external rotation. Ideally, if the child is not apprehensive, turn the child prone to assess the rotation with the hips extended. To do this, place one hand on the pelvis and rotate the hip internally and externally until you feel the pelvis move. Examine each hip individually. Estimate the degree of rotation and record it quickly on the examination paper to prevent confusion when documenting the examination in the medical record. Do one hip at a time and record the degree of internal and external rotation as you do the exam.

Tibial Torsion

Tibial torsion is most accurately evaluated with the patient prone on the examination table. It can be done at the same time as the hip rotation evaluation. However, I reserve this examination for older children, or children who are not fearful. With the child prone, flex the knee 90 degrees and imagine a line down the thigh and a line down the axis of the foot. This is the "thigh-foot-angle" and represents the amount of tibial torsion. For feet that turn inward as a result of twisting between the knee and the ankle (internal tibial torsion) this would be a negative thigh-foot-angle and is measured in degrees. Similarly, for feet that turn outward as a result of twisting of the tibia outward, the thigh-foot-angle would be a positive number.

With younger children, I do the examination on the parent's lap. Therefore, the degree of twisting of the tibia and the amount of twisting is assessed with the patient in a sitting or supine position. The children will be less fearful in this position, and it is easier to demonstrate to the parents why the child toes in. Show the parents the position of the leg between the knee and the ankle. Point the knee toward you and gently dorsiflex the foot to neutral. Show the parents that while the knee is facing you, the ankle joint is facing inward (internal tibial torsion) or outward (external tibial torsion). For a strong demonstration to the parents about the etiology, place the child in their in-utero position. Usually this will be with the hips externally rotated so the knees are facing outward, and the feet tucked in toward the midline. The tibia *has* to be twisted for the child to fit in the uterus; there is no in-utero position with the knees and feet straight ahead.

Remember that the child can also be packed in utero with the feet turned outward in the same direction as the knee and will be born with external tibial torsion. Most noticeable is when one leg has external tibial torsion and one has internal tibial torsion, giving a "windswept" appearance. The child can still be placed in this in-utero position to demonstrate to the parents.

Feet

Observe the feet separately from the tibia. From the bottom of the foot you will be able to see clearly if there is a "hooking" inward of the forefoot, giving it a bean shape. This is metatarsus adductus, or metatarsus varus. Assess how flexible it is by tickling the child or observing their spontaneous movements. If the child does not straighten it out spontaneously, stretch it and see if it is passively correctable.

Putting It All Together

Natural history: Many children when they start to walk have physiologic bow legs (genu varum). This is not a true varus. Confirm this by putting the patellae facing anteriorly and the bowing should be much less evident. They have soft tissue external rotation contractures of their hips from the in-utero positioning combined with internal tibial torsion. As a result, they walk with their knees turned outward and their feet straight ahead, giving an appearance of bow legs. This is one of the reasons toddlers look so cute running up and down your hallway in their diaper—every time they take a step, their knee flexes and looks like it is jutting out laterally. As the hips loosen up, usually by the age of 2 years, they walk with their knees forward, and now the internal tibial torsion is "uncovered" and they intoe. If you explain the natural history to the parents, they will be reassured, especially as time goes on and they see that the bowing is disappearing and the intoeing in is appearing as predicted. Over time, although it is slow, the tibial torsion and the femoral anteversion also correct. Beware, however, that all children do not fully correct these rotational "deformities." Family history and examining the parents can be useful in predicting how much the child will correct the intoeing by the time they reach adulthood.

By the time the children are age 3, they will typically have a true knock knee (genu valgum). If they have a combination of internal rotation of the hip (the typical child will sit in the "W" position easily) combined with external tibial torsion the knock knee appearance will be more pronounced. The typical physiologic genu valgum corrects spontaneously and the knees should be straight by about age 6 years.

Young babies who have external tibial torsion from their in-utero position, as typically seen with calcaneovalgus feet, will predictably outtoe when they start to walk. These children have external rotation contractures of their hips, but now combined with external tibial torsion. I describe it to parents as "hips like a baby, legs like an adult." As the hips loosen up and they walk with their knees straight ahead, their feet will also be straight ahead.

The children who have metatarsus adductus may spontaneously correct without treatment. It is usually detected at birth or shortly after birth. Often simple stretching is sufficient to fully correct the foot deformity. If it is rigid or severe, specific treatment may be needed.

Most intoeing and outtoeing, knock knees, and bowlegs are of concern in toddlers. However, older children may continue to intoe due to excessive internal rotation of their hips. If this is combined with internal tibial torsion that has persisted, then the intoeing may be very noticeable.

What Do You Do With an Abnormal Result?

First, determine if the history is consistent with a normal condition ("My child was so bow legged when he first started walking, and now he toes in."). If the examination is also consistent with normal intoeing and outtoeing, reassure the family. Keep a close eye on the child to be sure the condition is correcting and changing the way you expect.

ICD-9-CM Codes

736.89	Tibial torsion (internal and external)
736.41	Genu valgum
736.42	Genu varum
754.53	Metatarsus varus (adductus)
755.60	Unspecified/other congenital anomaly of LE

The American Academy of Pediatrics publishes a complete line of coding publications, including an annual edition of *Coding for Pediatrics*. For more information on these excellent resources, visit the American Academy of Pediatrics Online Bookstore at **www.aap.org/bookstore/.**

Most intoeing and outtoeing is normal. There is no predictable way to change the natural history, so simple examination and observation are indicated. There are exceptions to this, however. There are some children who reach early adolescence and they are unable to get their feet straight ahead due to femoral anteversion, or residual internal tibial torsion. Surgery may be indicated in these children. They should be referred to a pediatric orthopedist.

The adolescent who outtoes needs to be evaluated for a slipped capital femoral epiphysis. Do not overlook this diagnosis as the presenting complaints may be outtoeing and a limp. Adolescent children with genu varum should be referred to a pediatric orthopedist for diagnosis and treatment for possible adolescent Blounts.

MARCIA HERMAN-GIDDENS, PA, DrPH
PAUL B. KAPLOWITZ, MD

SEXUAL MATURITY STAGES

Sexual maturity staging is a standard assessment for normal growth and development. Identification of sexual maturity also is important in order to offer appropriate anticipatory guidance and to recognize problems related to pubertal abnormalities that need referral.

Why Is It Important to Assess Sexual Maturity Stages During the Physical Examination?

Children with early puberty may have problems coping with the physical and hormonal changes of puberty. Girls may have difficulty coping with early menses and boys may experience excessive libido. Early and rapidly progressive precocious puberty can sometimes result in adult short stature. Most cases of precocious puberty are idiopathic, but occasionally boys or girls with precocious puberty have intracranial abnormalities or adrenal or gonadal conditions that require intervention.

Children with delayed puberty may have conditions that require intervention. These children may be late maturers because of constitutional delayed puberty, for which there is often a positive family history. Other conditions that may need assessment or intervention include acquired gonadal failure, gonadal dysgenesis due to Turner syndrome, isolated gonadotropin deficiency, or decreased body fat due to exercise (particularly swimming, gymnastics, and ballet dancing), or anorexia nervosa.

The age of pubertal onset may be declining. Recent studies suggest that the age of onset of puberty is close to 1 year earlier in US girls than 30 years ago. Evidence as to whether a similar trend is occuring in boys is inconclusive at this time.

Early puberty may be a marker for environmental exposure to estrogen-like chemicals, known as endocrine disrupters, that may affect the reproductive axis. Currently no clear evidence exists that environmental chemicals are the major cause of earlier puberty in girls, but studies are ongoing.

Several studies suggest that earlier onset of puberty may be associated with being overweight in girls, and late onset may be associated with abnormal thinness or a very high sustained level of physical activity. With regard to boys, data on the relationship between overweight and earlier pubertal development are conflicting.

The issue of whether or not early puberty is associated with more frequent emotional problems is complex, and studies are conflicting. Many early-maturing children do well, but others show an increase in behavioral problems. Several papers report an increased incidence of psychopathology in young adults who started puberty at an early age. This suggests that early-maturing children need close monitoring of their physical and mental health.

Given the younger age of appearance of signs of puberty, anticipatory guidance for children and parents is even more important than it was in the past

Racial and ethnic differences in ages of achieving pubertal milestones vary. Results from the Pediatric Research in Office Settings study of puberty published in 1997 indicate that by the age of 8 to 9, approximately half of African-American girls and 15% of white girls will have some evidence of breast development, pubic hair growth, or both.

Girls: Median Age of Transition to Tanner Stages by Race/Ethnicity

Stage	White	African-American	Mexican-American
Pubic Hair			
2	10.57	9.43	10.39
3	11.8	10.57	11.70
4	13.00	11.90	13.19
5	16.33	14.70	16.30
Breast Development			
2	10.38	9.48	9.80
3	11.75	10.79	11.43
4	13.29	12.24	13.07
5	15.47	13.92	14.70

Source: Sun SS, Schubert CM, Cameron W, et al. National estimates of the timing of sexual maturation and racial differences among US children. *Pediatrics*. 2002:110;911–919.

Boys: Median Age of Transition to Tanner Stages by Race/Ethnicity

Stage	White	African-American	Mexican-American
Pubic Hair			
2	12	11.2	12.3
3	12.6	12.5	13.1
4	13.5	13.7	14.1
5	15.7	15.4	15.8
Genital Development			
2	10.1	9.5	10.4
3	12.4	11.8	12.5
4	13.5	13.4	13.7
5	15.9	14.9	15.7

Source: Herman-Giddens ME, Wang L, Koch G. Secondary sexual characteristics in boys. Estimates from the National Health and Nutrition Examination Survey III, 1988–1994. *Arch Pediatr Adolesc Med*. 2001:155.

Reliable data for American boys are not available for testicular growth. During the fourth grade (age 9), about 21% of African-American boys and 4% of white boys have at least Stage 2 pubic hair.

What Are the Stages of Sexual Maturity?

The system of sexual maturity rating most commonly used is based on the work of Marshall and Tanner. The stages are commonly referred to as the Tanner stages. This rating system has been widely used for decades in studies worldwide. There is no conventionally accepted scale for axillary hair development.

Pubic Hair: Male and Female

Pubic Hair Stage 1

Prepubertal. The vellus over the pubis is similar to that on the abdomen. This hair has not yet developed the characteristics of pubic hair.

Pubic Hair Stage 2

There is sparse growth of long, slightly pigmented downy hair, straight or only slightly curled, mainly at the base of the penis.

Pubic Hair Stage 3

The hair is considerably darker, coarser, and more curled. It is spread sparsely over the pubis.

Pubic Hair Stage 4

The hair is adult in type, but the area over which it is present is smaller than in most adults. It has not yet spread to the medial thighs or along the linea alba (in males).

Pubic Hair Stage 5

The hair is adult in quality and quantity and has the classical triangular distribution in females. It may spread to the medial surface of the thighs.

Breasts: Females

Breast Stage 1

There is no development. Only the nipple is elevated.

Breast Stage 2

The "breast bud" stage, the areola widens, slightly darkens, and elevates from the rest of the breast. A bud of glandular tissue is palpable below the nipple.

Breast Stage 3

The breast and areola further enlarge, presenting a rounded contour. There is no change of contour between the nipple and areola and the rest of the breast. The diameter of breast tissue is still smaller than in a mature breast.

Breast Stage 4

The breast continues to grow. The papilla and areola project to form a secondary mound above the rest of the breast.

Breast Stage 5

The mature adult stage. The secondary mound disappears. Some females never progress to Stage 5.

Genitals: Males

Genital Stage 1

Prepubertal. Penis, testes, and scrotum are about the same size and proportions as in early childhood. It is important to take into account whether the penis is uncircumsized when assessing penile growth, as the uncircumsized penis may appear larger than it really is.

Genital Stage 2

Only the testes and scrotum have begun to enlarge from the early childhood size. The penis is still prepubertal in appearance. The texture of the scrotal skin is beginning to become thinner and the skin appears redder due to increased vascularization.

Genital Stage 3

There is further growth of the testes and scrotum. The penis is also beginning to grow, mainly in length with some increase in breadth. It can be difficult to distinguish between Stages 2 and 3.

Genital Stage 4

The penis enlarges further in length and breadth and the glans becomes more prominent. The testes and scrotum are larger. There is further darkening of the scrotal skin.

Genital Stage 5

The penis, testes, and scrotum are adult in size and shape.

How Should You Perform Sexual Maturity Staging?

Pubic Hair Staging

- Ensure adequate lighting, and examine the genital area with the pants and underwear completely removed or lowered to the knees. This is especially true in girls, where the first pubic hair may initially be only along the labia.

- In assessing pubic hair do not confuse fine, light-colored hair in the genital area with pubic hair if it is similar to the hair found on other parts of the trunk or thighs.

- Familiarity with the pictures in standard texts (such as those shown in this chapter) is helpful but, in some children, the appearance does not match the pictures, as some children may be in between stages.

Breast Staging

- The Tanner method, which involves staging of breast development by **inspection alone** and comparing it with standard pictures found in many texts, needs to be supplemented by palpation for overweight girls.

  ▶ If further assessment is needed

    - Examine breast with patient in supine position. If the consistency under the areola is similar to peripheral tissue, it is likely adipose tissue. Breast tissue is firmer and discoid in shape.

    - In girls, the areola becomes thicker and darker with progressive exposure to estrogens.

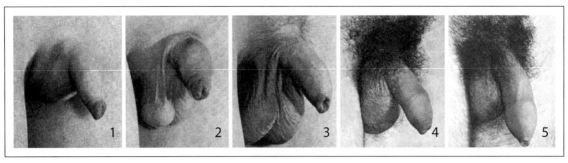

Boys stages of genital and pubic hair development.

Source: Reprinted of Elsevier from van Wieringen JC, Wafelbakker F, Verbrugge HP, De Haas JH. *Growth Diagrams 1965.* Groningen, The Netherlands: Wolters-Noordhoff; 1971. As included in Yen SSC, Jaffe RB, eds. *Reproductive Endocrinology: Physiology, Pathophysiology and Clinical Management.* 2nd ed. Philadelphia, PA: WB Saunders; 1978.

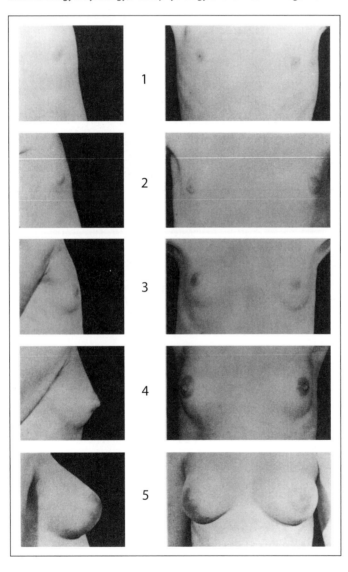

Girls stages of breast development

Source: Reprinted of Elsevier from van Wieringen JC, Wafelbakker F, Verbrugge HP, De Haas JH. Growth Diagrams 1965. Groningen, The Netherlands: Wolters-Noordhoff; 1971. As included in Yen SSC, Jaffe RB, eds. *Reproductive Endocrinology: Physiology, Pathophysiology and Clinical Management.* 2nd ed. Philadelphia, PA: WB Saunders; 1978.

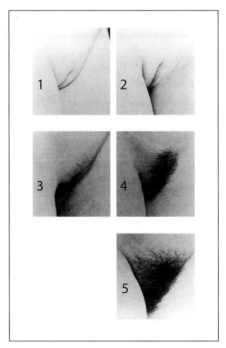

Girls stages of pubic hair growth.

Source: Reprinted of Elsevier from van Wieringen JC, Wafelbakker F, Verbrugge HP, De Haas JH. Growth Diagrams 1965. Groningen, The Netherlands: Wolters-Noordhoff; 1971. As included in Yen SSC, Jaffe RB, eds. *Reproductive Endocrinology: Physiology, Pathophysiology and Clinical Management.* 2nd ed. Philadelphia, PA: WB Saunders; 1978.

Male Genital Measurements

- The examiner should verify that the testes are descended and that the urethral opening is at the tip of the glans (ie, that the boy does not have hypospadius).

- In boys, the earliest and most reliable sign of pubertal development is enlargement of the testes, as it reflects increased secretion of the pituitary gonadotropins.

- Where further assessment is needed

  ▸ Testicular size can be assessed by comparing testes with beads of varying size developed by Prader, known as an orchidometer. The beads correspond to testicular volumes of 1 mL through 25 mL. Other methods of measurement include rulers, calipers, and ultrasound. Ultrasound is the most accurate measurement method.

  ▸ Another widely used method is to measure the greatest diameter by positioning the testis between the thumb, index, and middle finger and lining up a small ruler along the long axis of the testis.

  ▸ Prepubertal boys nearly always have a testicular length of 2.5 cm or less or volume of 4 mL or less. As puberty progresses, the increase in testicular size usually precedes the increase in penis size, and eventually reaches the adult size of 5.0 cm or 25 mL.

  ▸ Increasing penile length occurs later than initial growth of the testes.

  ▸ To measure penile length accurately, use either a ruler or a marked tongue blade pressed at the base of the penis while applying firm stretch to the penis itself.

  ▸ In normal prepubertal boys, the penile length is usually between 5 to 7 cm. A stretched length of 8 cm or greater indicates increased testosterone effect.

  ▸ The physical examination record should note for undescended testicles; penile abnormalities, such as chordee; hypospadias; or anomalous genital development.

    • Adrenal androgens, which cause pubic hair development, do not increase penile length.

What Should You Do With an Abnormal Result?

Precocious Puberty

General Observations

Any child with signs of early puberty should have growth carefully plotted. Pathology is not common but is more likely in those children showing clear acceleration of linear growth.

If the only abnormal finding is appearance of pubic hair (often accompanied by axillary hair and odor), the diagnosis is likely premature adrenarche, a benign normal variant due to an early increase in adrenal androgen secretion. It occurs more often in girls but is not infrequent in boys. The risk of pathology is low, and extensive hormone testing and x-ray evaluation are generally not needed, unless there is rapid progression of pubic hair and/or growth acceleration.

- Labs are of limited use in typical cases in which there is early appearance of pubic hair. Dehydroepiandorsterone sulfate (DHEA-S), 17-hydroxyprogesterone, testosterone, and bone age should be considered in higher-risk cases. Luteinizing hormone (LH), follicle stimulating hormone (FSH), and estradiol are of no value if there is no breast development.

Breast Development

Isolated breast development with normal growth starting before age 3 is most likely due to premature thelarche, another benign normal variant. These girls can be monitored by the primary care physician if there is no progression or referred to a specialist if there is rapid growth or significant increase in breast diameter over time.

Breast development starting between the ages of 3 and 7 should generally be referred if it has persisted for at least 6 months.

In girls ages 7 to 8, early breast development is most often found in normal girls who start to mature at the early end of the normal range. However, girls whose breast enlargement progresses rapidly (eg, already at Tanner 3 when first seen or rapidly increases to Tanner 3) are at higher risk of pathology.

- Useful labs for high-risk cases: LH, FSH, estradiol, and bone age

Nearly 20% of girls who start puberty before age 6 have abnormal brain magnetic resonance imaging findings (eg, a hypothalamic hamartoma [nonmalignant] or a glioma or astrocytoma), compared with about 2% of girls starting puberty between the ages of 6 and 8. The risk is much higher if there are new neurologic findings, such as visual abnormalities, severe and frequent headaches, or new onset of seizures.

Genital Development

Boys who have an increase in testicular and penile size before age 9 need to be referred for evaluation. Boys with a significant increase in penis size but not testicular enlargement may have congenital adrenal hyperplasia or a virilizing adrenal or testicular tumor. Boys with pubic hair only most likely have premature adrenarche; they should also be referred, though with less urgency.

- Useful labs if there is both testicular and penile growth: LH, FSH, testosterone, and bone age

- Useful labs if there is increased penile growth but prepubertal testes: testosterone, 17-hydroxyprogesterone, DHEA-S, and bone age

Delayed Puberty

Girls who have not started having breast enlargement by age 13 and boys who have not started having penile and testicular enlargement by age 14 are, by definition, delayed and need to be evaluated and appropriately managed.

- Useful labs: LH, FSH (will be elevated in gonadal failure), testosterone (in boys), estradiol (in girls), and bone age

A child with delayed puberty and significant slowing of growth may need to be evaluated for growth hormone and possibly other pituitary hormone deficiencies, as well as other chronic diseases (eg, gastrointestinal, renal, cardiac, pulmonary).

What Results Should You Document?

Record Tanner staging in the chart at all routine health supervision visits. For patients showing signs of early or delayed pubertal maturation, it may be helpful in these cases to see the child every 6 months rather than yearly, before deciding if a referral to an endocrinologist is needed.

Document lab tests and x-rays ordered, and results, as well as the follow-up plan.

If the child is referred to a specialist for further evaluation, be certain to give a copy of the results of any hormone testing or x-rays done as well as the growth chart to the parents to take to the appointment.

Be certain to send full evaluation testing on growth chart to referral source.

ICD-9-CM Codes	
259.0	Delayed puberty
259.1	Precocious puberty, premature adrenarche; premature thelarche

The American Academy of Pediatrics publishes a complete line of coding publications, including an annual edition of *Coding for Pediatrics*. For more information on these excellent resources, visit the American Academy of Pediatrics Online Bookstore at **www.aap.org/bookstore/**.

Resources

Evidenced-based Guidelines

Kaplowitz PB, Oberfield SE; Drug and Therapeutics and Executive Committee of the Lawson Wilkins Pediatric Endocrine Society. Reexamination of the age limit for defining when puberty is precocious in girls in the United States: implications for evaluation and treatment. *Pediatrics*. 1999;104:936–941

Books

Herman-Giddens ME, Bourdony CJ. *Assessment of Sexual Maturity Stages in Boys*. Elk Grove Village, IL: Pediatric Research in Office Settings, American Academy of Pediatrics; 2005

Herman-Giddens ME, Bourdony CJ. *Assessment of Sexual Maturity Stages in Girls*. Elk Grove Village, IL: Pediatric Research in Office Settings, American Academy of Pediatrics; 1995

- *Abduction/adduction:* This maneuver is especially important in toddlers. Developmental dysplasia of the hip (DDH) may have no obvious sign other than limited hip abduction unilaterally and/or bilateral waddling gait.

With the child supine on the examination table, the knees are brought maximally away from midline both at full hip extension and at 90 degrees' hip flexion. Measure abduction by recording the angle subtended between the midline axis and the femur at the extremes of abduction. Adduction is measured similarly in hip extension but with the knees brought toward and past midline.

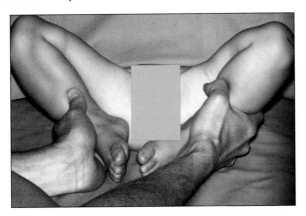

Conduct a provocative test

- *Trendelenburg sign:* Intra-articular hip pathology frequently induces weakness in hip abduction. Hip abduction raises the joint reactive forces across the painful hip, and is avoided. Weakness will be evident when the patient stands on the ipsilateral lower limb. A positive Trendelenburg sign is defined as the contralateral pelvis dropping below level, or the patient leaning over the painful hip for balance. Compare side to side. Single-leg stance on the normal hip with normal abductor strength will maintain a level pelvis.

- *Barlow provocative test:* This maneuver is intended to screen an infant (0–3 months of age) for DDH. With the infant supine on a firm surface and sufficiently calm, flex the both hips to 90 degrees (thighs will be perpendicular to the trunk if the knees are also at 90-degree flexion). Hold the infant's thighs with thumbs medially and fingers laterally. The infant's knees are nested in the examiners first web space. Apply posterior (downward) pressure. A positive Barlow test will yield a clunk sensation as the femoral head

subluxes or dislocates from the acetabulum. A negative test should yield firm, smooth resistance without yield or clunk.

- *Ortolani test:* Also for DDH screening, this test is performed in infants 0 to 3 months of age. Hold hips as in Barlow, grasping knee between thumb and fingers, but place the tip of (second or third digit) finger(s) over the infant's greater trochanters. Abduct hips with the thumbs and simultaneously apply medial and anterior pressure with the long fingers. A positive test will reduce the femoral heads into the acetabulum during abduction.

Perform a Knee Examination

Observe. With the child standing in a 2-leg stance, observe the overall alignment of the lower limbs. When the ankles are centered under the anterior-superior iliac spines, the patella should be roughly vertically aligned between them. The normal degree of coronal plane angulation across the knee will vary with age. Infants are born with physiologic varus or bow-legged alignment of their lower extremities. This corrects to neutral alignment by 18 to 24 months of age. Maximal valgus, or knock-kneed alignment, is characteristic of 3- to 5-year-olds. Normal adult alignment of 7 degrees of valgus between the tibia and the femur is reached by early school age. Watch the child walk and look for a lateral thrust of the knee, or an opening up of the knee into a more varus position. This may indicate that the bowing is not physiologic.

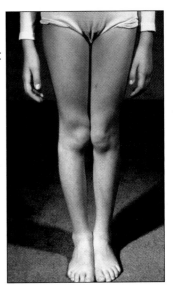

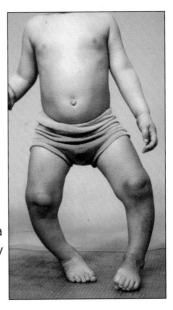

Palpate. Differentiate effusion from generalized swelling by the presence of a fluid wave or by shifting of the area of maximal swelling with variously applied manual pressure over bulging areas of the joint capsule. Tenderness of the knee just proximal to the tibial plateau, at the joint line (laterally or medially), is suggestive of (lateral or medial) meniscal pathology. Prominence or tenderness of the tibial tubercle suggests a diagnosis of Osgood-Schlatter disease.

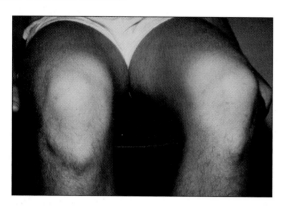

Assess. Knee motion ranges from full extension, where the tibia and femur are parallel, to full flexion, where the heel touches the ipsilateral buttocks.

To evaluate genu varum (bow legs) or genu valgum (knock knees), the child should be supine on the examination table with the knees and hips extended and adducted until the limbs touch.

If the knees touch first, measure the distance between the medial malleoli of the ankles (intermalleolar distance). This is a quantitative measure of clinical valgus. If the ankles approximate first, the distance between the medial femoral condyles (intercondylar distance) is the quantification of genu varum.

If the child is apprehensive, the child can be examined in the parent's lap: Child and parent will be facing examiner with child seated in lap. Hips and knees are flexed 90 degrees with knees facing examiner. If there is internal tibial torsion, feet will cross. If bowing (or valgus) is no longer present, the condition is likely physiologic.

To evaluate Q-angle: With the child lying supine, but with the knee flexed 30 degrees, the angle between a line connecting the anterior superior iliac spine and the center of the patella and a line from the center of the patella to the tibial tubercle (the insertion of the patella tendon).

This angle is normally 12 degrees with the apex toward the midline. Increases in this angle may be associated with patellofemoral instability.

Scales or Tools

No specific grades or tools exist for these examinations. Symmetry is more important than meeting a set expected range of motion.

What Should You Do With an Abnormal Result?

For hip abnormalities in an infant, maintain a low threshold. Refer the infant for plain films (generally after 4 months of age) of the hips or for ultrasonography (usually done in the first 2–4 months, if a specialist with experience in this technique is available in your medical care system). Make the referral to the orthopedic surgeon who cares for children's orthopedic problems in your referral system. This specialist may be a general orthopedic surgeon or a pediatric orthopedic surgeon.

Consider skeletal dysplasia in any child with genu varum or valgus deformities who has poor linear growth. If the child is bow legged, and it is getting worse over time, consider rickets (obtain a dietary history; examine wrists for metaphyseal flaring; examine ribs for beading; and obtain radiographs, calcium, phosphorus, alkaline phosphatase, and 25 OH vitamin D).

Infantile Blount's disease, or tibia vara, must be considered in children who walk early and have an increasing or persistent varus deformity at 2 1/2 years, especially with lateral thrust on weight bearing. This is a radiographic diagnosis and requires consultation from a pediatric orthopedist.

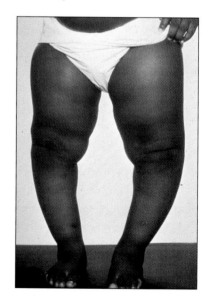

For patients who have a single kidney or a single functioning kidney, the athlete needs individual assessment for contact, collision, and limited-contact sports and a clear discussion about the risks of participation in sports and recreational activities that may have incidental or deliberate contact. Protective equipment may reduce risk of injury to the remaining kidney sufficiently to allow participation in most sports, providing such equipment remains in place during activity.

For athletes who have one paired organ, every effort should be made for some type of sports participation, with protective gear if necessary.

What Should You Do With an Abnormal Result?

The results of your history and examination will lead to 1 of 3 categories for sports participation: **cleared, not cleared,** and **in need of further evaluation.** It is quite straightforward when an athlete is cleared. The confusing area is when a student athlete is temporarily not cleared or is in need of further evaluation. This category may result from an injury (eg, a fracture or recent surgery) or medical condition (infectious mononucleosis or concussion).

In these circumstances, it is extremely important to have a coordinated approach with the team coach, family, and athlete.

What Results Should You Document?

The patient's health record and school forms need to indicate the student's participation or restrictions.

Resources

Articles

American Academy of Pediatrics Committee on Sports Medicine and Fitness. Protective eyewear for young athletes. *Pediatrics.* 2004;113:619–622

Graham TP Jr, Bricker JT, James FW, Strong WB. 26th Bethesda Conference: recommendations for determining eligibility for competition in athletes with cardiovascular abnormalities. *Med Sci Sports Exerc.* 1994;26(10 suppl):S223–S283

Grinsell MM, Showalter S, Gordon KA, Norwood VF. Single kidney and sports participation: perception versus reality. *Pediatrics.* 2006;118;1019–1027

Maron BJ, Thompson PD, Ackerman MJ, et al. Recommendations and considerations related to preparticipation screening for cardiovascular abnormalities in competitive athletes: 2007 update: a scientific statement from the American Heart Association Council on Nutrition, Physical Activity, and Metabolism: endorsed by the American College of Cardiology Foundation. *Circulation.* 2007;115:1643

McCory P, Johnston K, Meeuwisse W, et al. Summary and agreement statement of the 2nd International Conference on Concussion in Sport, Prague 2004. *Br J Sports Med.* 2005;39:196–204

Mitten MJ, Maron BJ, Zipes DP. Task Force 12: legal aspects of the 36th Bethesda Conference recommendations. *J Am Coll Cardiol.* 2005;45:1373–75

Rice SG; American Academy of Pediatrics Council on Sports Medicine and Fitness. Medical conditions affecting sports participation. *Pediatrics.* 2008;121;841–848

Schluep C, ed. Burners (brachial plexus injuries): sports medicine guidelines. In: Klossner D, NCAA Staff. *NCAA Sports Medicine Handbook 2003–2004.* Indianapolis, IN: National Collegiate Athletic Association; 2007:51

Reference

1. American Academy of Family Physicians, American Academy of Pediatrics, American College of Sports Medicine, American Medical Society for Sports Medicine, American Orthopaedic Society for Sports Medicine. and American Osteopathic Academy of Sports Medicine, the Preparticipation Physical Evaluation. 4th ed. Elk Grove Village, IL: American Academy of Pediatrics; 2010

■ PREPARTICIPATION PHYSICAL EVALUATION
HISTORY FORM

(Note: This form is to be filled out by the patient and parent prior to seeing the physician. The physician should keep this form in the chart.)

Date of Exam _____

Name _____ Date of birth _____

Sex _____ Age _____ Grade _____ School _____ Sport(s) _____

Medicines and Allergies: Please list all of the prescription and over-the-counter medicines and supplements (herbal and nutritional) that you are currently taking

_____
_____

Do you have any allergies? ☐ Yes ☐ No   If yes, please identify specific allergy below.
☐ Medicines   ☐ Pollens   ☐ Food   ☐ Stinging Insects

Explain "Yes" answers below. Circle questions you don't know the answers to.

GENERAL QUESTIONS	Yes	No
1. Has a doctor ever denied or restricted your participation in sports for any reason?		
2. Do you have any ongoing medical conditions? If so, please identify below: ☐ Asthma ☐ Anemia ☐ Diabetes ☐ Infections Other: _____		
3. Have you ever spent the night in the hospital?		
4. Have you ever had surgery?		

HEART HEALTH QUESTIONS ABOUT YOU	Yes	No
5. Have you ever passed out or nearly passed out DURING or AFTER exercise?		
6. Have you ever had discomfort, pain, tightness, or pressure in your chest during exercise?		
7. Does your heart ever race or skip beats (irregular beats) during exercise?		
8. Has a doctor ever told you that you have any heart problems? If so, check all that apply: ☐ High blood pressure ☐ A heart murmur ☐ High cholesterol ☐ A heart infection ☐ Kawasaki disease Other: _____		
9. Has a doctor ever ordered a test for your heart? (For example, ECG/EKG, echocardiogram)		
10. Do you get lightheaded or feel more short of breath than expected during exercise?		
11. Have you ever had an unexplained seizure?		
12. Do you get more tired or short of breath more quickly than your friends during exercise?		

HEART HEALTH QUESTIONS ABOUT YOUR FAMILY	Yes	No
13. Has any family member or relative died of heart problems or had an unexpected or unexplained sudden death before age 50 (including drowning, unexplained car accident, or sudden infant death syndrome)?		
14. Does anyone in your family have hypertrophic cardiomyopathy, Marfan syndrome, arrhythmogenic right ventricular cardiomyopathy, long QT syndrome, short QT syndrome, Brugada syndrome, or catecholaminergic polymorphic ventricular tachycardia?		
15. Does anyone in your family have a heart problem, pacemaker, or implanted defibrillator?		
16. Has anyone in your family had unexplained fainting, unexplained seizures, or near drowning?		

BONE AND JOINT QUESTIONS	Yes	No
17. Have you ever had an injury to a bone, muscle, ligament, or tendon that caused you to miss a practice or a game?		
18. Have you ever had any broken or fractured bones or dislocated joints?		
19. Have you ever had an injury that required x-rays, MRI, CT scan, injections, therapy, a brace, a cast, or crutches?		
20. Have you ever had a stress fracture?		
21. Have you ever been told that you have or have you had an x-ray for neck instability or atlantoaxial instability? (Down syndrome or dwarfism)		
22. Do you regularly use a brace, orthotics, or other assistive device?		
23. Do you have a bone, muscle, or joint injury that bothers you?		
24. Do any of your joints become painful, swollen, feel warm, or look red?		
25. Do you have any history of juvenile arthritis or connective tissue disease?		

MEDICAL QUESTIONS	Yes	No
26. Do you cough, wheeze, or have difficulty breathing during or after exercise?		
27. Have you ever used an inhaler or taken asthma medicine?		
28. Is there anyone in your family who has asthma?		
29. Were you born without or are you missing a kidney, an eye, a testicle (males), your spleen, or any other organ?		
30. Do you have groin pain or a painful bulge or hernia in the groin area?		
31. Have you had infectious mononucleosis (mono) within the last month?		
32. Do you have any rashes, pressure sores, or other skin problems?		
33. Have you had a herpes or MRSA skin infection?		
34. Have you ever had a head injury or concussion?		
35. Have you ever had a hit or blow to the head that caused confusion, prolonged headache, or memory problems?		
36. Do you have a history of seizure disorder?		
37. Do you have headaches with exercise?		
38. Have you ever had numbness, tingling, or weakness in your arms or legs after being hit or falling?		
39. Have you ever been unable to move your arms or legs after being hit or falling?		
40. Have you ever become ill while exercising in the heat?		
41. Do you get frequent muscle cramps when exercising?		
42. Do you or someone in your family have sickle cell trait or disease?		
43. Have you had any problems with your eyes or vision?		
44. Have you had any eye injuries?		
45. Do you wear glasses or contact lenses?		
46. Do you wear protective eyewear, such as goggles or a face shield?		
47. Do you worry about your weight?		
48. Are you trying to or has anyone recommended that you gain or lose weight?		
49. Are you on a special diet or do you avoid certain types of foods?		
50. Have you ever had an eating disorder?		
51. Do you have any concerns that you would like to discuss with a doctor?		
FEMALES ONLY		
52. Have you ever had a menstrual period?		
53. How old were you when you had your first menstrual period?		
54. How many periods have you had in the last 12 months?		

Explain "yes" answers here

_____
_____
_____
_____
_____
_____

I hereby state that, to the best of my knowledge, my answers to the above questions are complete and correct.

Signature of athlete _____ Signature of parent/guardian _____ Date _____

9-2681/0410

THE ATHLETE WITH SPECIAL NEEDS: SUPPLEMENTAL HISTORY FORM

Date of Exam _____

Name _____ Date of birth _____

Sex _____ Age _____ Grade _____ School _____ Sport(s) _____

	Yes	No
1. Type of disability		
2. Date of disability		
3. Classification (if available)		
4. Cause of disability (birth, disease, accident/trauma, other)		
5. List the sports you are interested in playing		
6. Do you regularly use a brace, assistive device, or prosthetic?		
7. Do you use any special brace or assistive device for sports?		
8. Do you have any rashes, pressure sores, or any other skin problems?		
9. Do you have a hearing loss? Do you use a hearing aid?		
10. Do you have a visual impairment?		
11. Do you use any special devices for bowel or bladder function?		
12. Do you have burning or discomfort when urinating?		
13. Have you had autonomic dysreflexia?		
14. Have you ever been diagnosed with a heat-related (hyperthermia) or cold-related (hypothermia) illness?		
15. Do you have muscle spasticity?		
16. Do you have frequent seizures that cannot be controlled by medication?		

Explain "yes" answers here

_____

_____

_____

_____

_____

Please indicate if you have ever had any of the following.

	Yes	No
Atlantoaxial instability		
X-ray evaluation for atlantoaxial instability		
Dislocated joints (more than one)		
Easy bleeding		
Enlarged spleen		
Hepatitis		
Osteopenia or osteoporosis		
Difficulty controlling bowel		
Difficulty controlling bladder		
Numbness or tingling in arms or hands		
Numbness or tingling in legs or feet		
Weakness in arms or hands		
Weakness in legs or feet		
Recent change in coordination		
Recent change in ability to walk		
Spina bifida		
Latex allergy		

Explain "yes" answers here

_____

_____

_____

_____

_____

I hereby state that, to the best of my knowledge, my answers to the above questions are complete and correct.

Signature of athlete _____ Signature of parent/guardian _____ Date _____

PHYSICAL EXAMINATION

■ PREPARTICIPATION PHYSICAL EVALUATION
PHYSICAL EXAMINATION FORM

Name _____ Date of birth _____

PHYSICIAN REMINDERS
1. Consider additional questions on more sensitive issues
   - Do you feel stressed out or under a lot of pressure?
   - Do you ever feel sad, hopeless, depressed, or anxious?
   - Do you feel safe at your home or residence?
   - Have you ever tried cigarettes, chewing tobacco, snuff, or dip?
   - During the past 30 days, did you use chewing tobacco, snuff, or dip?
   - Do you drink alcohol or use any other drugs?
   - Have you ever taken anabolic steroids or used any other performance supplement?
   - Have you ever taken any supplements to help you gain or lose weight or improve your performance?
   - Do you wear a seat belt, use a helmet, and use condoms?
2. Consider reviewing questions on cardiovascular symptoms (questions 5–14).

EXAMINATION			
Height	Weight	☐ Male ☐ Female	
BP ___ / ___ (___ / ___) Pulse ___		Vision R 20/___ L 20/___	Corrected ☐ Y ☐ N

MEDICAL	NORMAL	ABNORMAL FINDINGS
Appearance • Marfan stigmata (kyphoscoliosis, high-arched palate, pectus excavatum, arachnodactyly, arm span > height, hyperlaxity, myopia, MVP, aortic insufficiency)		
Eyes/ears/nose/throat • Pupils equal • Hearing		
Lymph nodes		
Heart [a] • Murmurs (auscultation standing, supine, +/- Valsalva) • Location of point of maximal impulse (PMI)		
Pulses • Simultaneous femoral and radial pulses		
Lungs		
Abdomen		
Genitourinary (males only) [b]		
Skin • HSV, lesions suggestive of MRSA, tinea corporis		
Neurologic [c]		
MUSCULOSKELETAL		
Neck		
Back		
Shoulder/arm		
Elbow/forearm		
Wrist/hand/fingers		
Hip/thigh		
Knee		
Leg/ankle		
Foot/toes		
Functional • Duck-walk, single leg hop		

[a]Consider ECG, echocardiogram, and referral to cardiology for abnormal cardiac history or exam.
[b]Consider GU exam if in private setting. Having third party present is recommended.
[c]Consider cognitive evaluation or baseline neuropsychiatric testing if a history of significant concussion.

☐ Cleared for all sports without restriction

☐ Cleared for all sports without restriction with recommendations for further evaluation or treatment for _____

_____

☐ Not cleared
   ☐ Pending further evaluation
   ☐ For any sports
   ☐ For certain sports _____
   Reason _____
Recommendations _____

I have examined the above-named student and completed the preparticipation physical evaluation. The athlete does not present apparent clinical contraindications to practice and participate in the sport(s) as outlined above. A copy of the physical exam is on record in my office and can be made available to the school at the request of the parents. If conditions arise after the athlete has been cleared for participation, the physician may rescind the clearance until the problem is resolved and the potential consequences are completely explained to the athlete (and parents/guardians).

Name of physician (print/type) _____ Date _____
Address _____ Phone _____
Signature of physician _____, MD or DO

9-2681/0410

CLEARANCE FORM

Name _____ Sex ☐ M ☐ F Age _____ Date of birth _____

☐ Cleared for all sports without restriction

☐ Cleared for all sports without restriction with recommendations for further evaluation or treatment for _____

_____

☐ Not cleared

      ☐ Pending further evaluation

      ☐ For any sports

      ☐ For certain sports _____

      Reason _____

Recommendations _____

_____

_____

_____

_____

_____

I have examined the above-named student and completed the preparticipation physical evaluation. The athlete does not present apparent clinical contraindications to practice and participate in the sport(s) as outlined above. A copy of the physical exam is on record in my office and can be made available to the school at the request of the parents. If conditions arise after the athlete has been cleared for participation, the physician may rescind the clearance until the problem is resolved and the potential consequences are completely explained to the athlete (and parents/guardians).

Name of physician (print/type) _____ Date _____

Address _____ Phone _____

Signature of physician _____, MD or DO

EMERGENCY INFORMATION

Allergies _____

_____

_____

_____

_____

Other information _____

_____

_____

_____

_____

_____

_____

_____

SCREENING

S creening occurs at each Bright Futures health supervision visit. Certain screenings are universal (ie, they are applied to each child at a particular visit). For example, all children at the 1-year visit are screened for lead exposure. Other screenings are selective (ie, they occur only if a risk assessment is positive). For example, a child will receive a tuberculin skin test at the 7-year visit if he or she answers positively on risk screening questions.

The chapters in this section of the book were selected because they provide important "how-to" information to guide health care professionals. The **Immunizations, Newborn Screening, and Capillary Blood Tests** chapter provides up-to-date information on all the immunization schedules. Ensuring that all children's and adolescents' immunizations are complete is an essential element of preventive health services and a key component of each Bright Futures visit.

SCREENING

JOHN KNIGHT, MD
TIMOTHY ROBERTS, MD, MPH
JOY GABRIELLI, MD
SHARI VAN HOOK, MPH

ADOLESCENT ALCOHOL AND SUBSTANCE USE AND ABUSE

Why Is It Important to Screen for Adolescent Alcohol and Substance Use?

Alcohol and substance use is associated with deaths, injuries, and health problems among US teenagers. Use is associated with leading causes of death, including unintentional injuries (eg, motor vehicle crashes), homicides, and suicides. More than 30% of all deaths from injuries can be directly linked to alcohol. Substance use also is associated with a wide range of non-lethal but serious health problems, including school failure, respiratory diseases, and high-risk sexual behaviors.

Alcohol and substance use is common among adolescents. Studies show that 46% of adolescents have tried alcohol by eighth grade, and by senior year in high school 77% of adolescents have begun to drink. Moreover, 20% of eighth graders and 58% of seniors have been drunk.

Adolescents have recently reported increasing misuse of prescription drugs, including psychostimulant medications and oral opioid analgesics.

Two factors can predict increases in the prevalence of use of specific illicit drugs.

- An increase in the perceived availability of the drug

- A decrease in the perceived risk of harm associated with use of the drug

Misuse of alcohol and drugs is found among all demographic subgroups. Higher risk of misuse is associated with being male, white, and from middle to upper socioeconomic status families.

Early age of first use of alcohol and drugs can increase the risk of developing a substance use disorder during later life.

Recurrent drunkenness, recurrent cannabis use, or any use of drugs other than cannabis are not normative behaviors, and health care practitioners should always consider them serious risks. However, experimentation with alcohol or cannabis or getting drunk once can arguably be considered developmentally normative behaviors.

When Should You Evaluate an Adolescent's Alcohol or Substance Use?

Substance use should be evaluated as part of an age-appropriate comprehensive history. Reviewing the adolescent's environment can identify risk and protective factors for the development of alcohol or drug abuse.

Risk Factors

- A family history of substance abuse or mood disorders. One in 5 children grows up in a household where someone abuses alcohol or other drugs. Substance use by a family member is associated with higher rates of substance use in adolescents.

- Poor parental supervision and household disruption are associated with involvement in substance use and other risk behaviors.

- Low academic achievement and/or academic aspirations.

- Untreated attention-deficit disorder (ADD) and attention-deficit/hyperactivity disorder (ADHD).

SCREENING

- Perceived peer acceptance of substance use and substance use in peers.

Protective Factors

- Parents who set clear rules and enforce them.

- Eating meals together as a family.

- Parents who regularly talk with their children about the dangers of alcohol and drug use.

- Having a parent in recovery.

- Involvement in church, synagogue, or community programs.

- Opportunities for prosocial involvement in the community, adequate community resources.

How Should You Evaluate an Adolescent's Alcohol or Substance Use?

Use Informal Methods

- Ask about alcohol and substance use. Many adolescents do not discuss their substance use with their physician. The most common reason given for not discussing substance use during a clinic visit was never being asked. Evidence shows that 65% of adolescents report a desire to discuss substance use during clinic visits.

- Begin with open-ended questions about substance use at home and school and by peers before progressing to open-ended questions about personal use. Two questions that can readily screen for the need to ask further questions include

  Have you ever had an alcoholic drink?

  Have you ever used marijuana or any other drug to get high?[1]

- Recognize the importance and complexity of confidentiality issues. Providing a place where the adolescent can speak confidentially is associated with greater disclosure of risk behavior involvement. Time alone with the physician during the clinic visit is associated with greater disclosure of sensitive information.

At the same time, the confidentiality of your conversation is limited by an adolescent's reports of threat to self, threat to others, and abuse. After reviewing the severity of an adolescent's substance use, you can judge the seriousness of a threat to self.

Discuss the need to disclose sensitive information with the adolescent before disclosing to parents or other people (treatment specialists, for example).

Use Screening Tools

The evidence supporting screening for substance misuse in adolescents is Type IV (Expert Opinion) because no clinical trials support the efficacy of screening during clinical encounters. However, several tools are available, and the CRAFFT screener (Boxes 1 and 2) has high sensitivities and specificities for identifying a diagnosis of substance problem use, abuse, or dependence.[2]

Consider using a pen and paper (GAPS screening tool, Problem-Oriented Screening Instrument for Teenagers [POSIT]) or computerized screening tool before clinic appointments.

Or use a structured interview designed to detect serious substance use in adolescents, such as the CRAFFT screener.

A positive CRAFFT should be followed by a more comprehensive alcohol and drug use history, including age of first use; current pattern of use (quantity and frequency); impact on physical and emotional health, school, and family; and other negative consequences from use (eg, legal problems).

Taking a good substance use history begins the process of therapeutic intervention. Helpful questions include

- What's the worst thing that ever happened to you while you were using alcohol or drugs?

- Have you ever regretted something that happened when you were drinking or taking drugs?

- Do your parents know about your alcohol and drug use? If so, how do they feel about it? If not, how do you think they would feel about it?

- Do you have any younger brothers or sisters? What do (or would) they think about your alcohol and drug use?

The assessment should also include a screening for co-occurring mental disorders and parent/sibling alcohol and drug use.

Box 1. The CRAFFT Screening Interview

Begin: "I'm going to ask you a few questions that I ask all my patients. Please be honest. I will keep your answers confidential."

Part A

During the PAST 12 MONTHS, did you:	No	Yes
1. Drink any alcohol (more than a few sips)? (Do not count sips of alcohol taken during family or religious events.)	☐	☐
2. Smoke any marijuana or hashish?	☐	☐
3. Use *anything else* to *get high*? ("anything else" includes illegal drugs, over the counter and prescription drugs, and things that you sniff or "huff")	☐	☐

For clinic use only: Did the patient answer "yes" to any questions in Part A?

No ☐   Yes ☐
↓   ↓
Ask CAR question only, then stop   Ask all 6 CRAFFT questions in Part B

Part B

	No	Yes
1. Have you ever ridden in a **CAR** driven by someone (including yourself) who was "high" or had been using alcohol or drugs?	☐	☐
2. Do you ever use alcohol or drugs to **RELAX,** feel better about yourself, or fit in?	☐	☐
3. Do you ever use alcohol or drugs while you are by yourself, or **ALONE**?	☐	☐
4. Do you ever **FORGET** things you did while using alcohol or drugs?	☐	☐
5. Do your **FAMILY** or **FRIENDS** ever tell you that you should cut down on your drinking or drug use?	☐	☐
6. Have you ever gotten into **TROUBLE** while you were using alcohol or drugs?	☐	☐

SCREENING

105

Table 2. The CRAFFT Screening Interview Scoring Instructions: For Clinic Staff Use Only

CRAFFT Scoring: Each "yes" response in **Part B** scores 1 point.
A total score of 2 or higher is a positive screen, indicating a need for additional assessment.

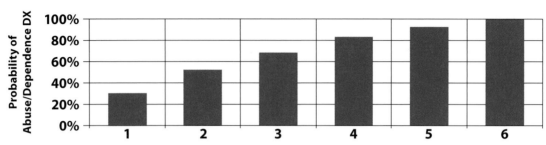

Probability of Substance Abuse/Dependence Diagnosis Based on CRAFFT Score[1,2]

DSM-IV Diagnostic Criteria[3] (Abbreviated)

Substance Abuse (1 or more of the following):

- Use causes failure to fulfill obligations at work, school, or home
- Recurrent use in hazardous situations (e.g. driving)
- Recurrent legal problems
- Continued use despite recurrent problems

Substance Dependence (3 or more of the following):

- Tolerance
- Withdrawal
- Substance taken in larger amount or over longer period of time than planned
- Unsuccessful efforts to cut down or quit
- Great deal of time spent to obtain substance or recover from effect
- Important activities given up because of substance
- Continued use despite harmful consequences

© Children's Hospital Boston, 2009. This form may be reproduced in its exact form for use in clinical settings, courtesy of the Center for Adolescent Substance Abuse Research, Children's Hospital Boston, 300 Longwood Ave, Boston, MA 02115, U.S.A., (617) 355-5433, www.ceasar.org.

References:

1. Knight JR, Shrier LA, Bravender TD, Farrell M, Vander Bilt J, Shaffer HJ. A new brief screen for adolescent substance abuse. *Arch Pediatr Adolesc Med.* 1999;153(6):591–596

2. Knight JR, Sherritt L, Shrier LA, Harris SK, Chang G. Validity of the CRAFFT substance abuse screening test among adolescent clinic patients. *Arch Pediatr Adolesc Med.* 2002;156(6):607–614

3. American Psychiatric Association. *Diagnostic and Statistical Manual of Mental Disorders.* 4th ed. Text rev. Washington, DC: American Psychiatric Association; 2000.

Rahdert ER, ed. *The Adolescent Assessment/Referral System Manual*. Washington, DC: US Department of Health and Human Services (PHS) Alcohol, Drug Abuse, and Mental Health Administration; 1991. DHHS Publication. No. (ADM) 91-1735

Schydlower M, ed. *Substance Abuse: A Guide for Health Professionals*. 2nd ed. Elk Grove Village, IL: American Academy of Pediatrics; 2002

Substance Abuse and Mental Health Services Administration. *The Relationship Between Mental Health and Substance Abuse Among Adolescents*. Rockville, MD: Substance Abuse and Mental Health Services Administration, Office of Applied Studies; 1999. OAS Analytic Series #9, DHHS Publication No. (SMA) 99-3286

Resources for Parents

Web Sites

A Family Guide To Keeping Youth Mentally Health and Drug Free: http://family.samhsa.gov/

Mothers Against Drunk Driving: http://www.madd.org

Parents: The Anti-Drug: http://www.theantidrug.com/

Partnership for a Drug Free America: http://www.drugfreeamerica.org

Books

Keeping Your Kids Drug Free: A How-to Guide for Parents and Caregivers: available online at http://ncadi.samhsa.gov/govpubs/phd884/

Keeping Youth Drug Free: available online at: http://ncadi.samhsa.gov/govpubs/phd711/

Treating Teens: A Guide to Adolescent Drug Programs. Washington, DC: Drug Strategies; 2003. http://www.eric.ed.gov/ERICDocs/data/ericdocs2sql/content_storage_01/0000019b/80/1a/da/9a.pdf

Resources for Teens

Web Sites

Check Yourself: http://www.checkyourself.com

NIDA for Teens (National Institute on Drug Abuse): http://www.teens.drugabuse.gov/

Students Against Destructive Decisions: http://saddonline.com

What's Driving You? http://www.whatsdrivingyou.org/

References

1. Levy S, Knight JR. Office management of substance use. *Adolesc Health Update*. 2003;15:1–11

2. Knight JR, Sherritt L, Shrier LA, Harris SK, Chang G. Validity of the CRAFFT substance abuse screening test among adolescent clinic patients. *Arch Pediatr Adolesc Med*. 2002;156:607–614

3. Ewing JA. Detecting alcoholism: the CAGE questionnaire. *JAMA*. 1984;252:1905–1907

SUSAN M. YUSSMAN, MD, MPH

CERVICAL DYSPLASIA

Why Is It Important to Screen for Cervical Dysplasia?

Cervical cancer can be prevented. Cervical cancer is the second most common cancer in women worldwide. Routine Papanicolaou (Pap) tests can detect most pre-invasive lesions before they progress to cancer. Since routine Pap screening began in the 1950s, the incidence of cervical cancer has decreased more than 70% in the United States.

Risk factors for developing cervical cancer include, but are not limited to, persistent infection with high-risk human papillomavirus (HPV) type, impaired immunity, cigarette smoking, increased parity, and prolonged oral contraceptive use.

Screening and observation have increased in importance because of changes to treatment guidelines for cervical dysplasia. These guidelines, updated in 2009, take into consideration that in adolescents with normal immunity, cervical cell abnormalities are mostly transient and regress spontaneously. In the US, only .1% of cases of cervical cancer occur before age 21, with less than 15 cases annually of invasive cancer in teens ages 15–19 years.

Therefore, there has been a shift from aggressive therapy of LSIL with colposcopy to closely monitored observation. Likewise, HPV DNA testing is now recommended as an adjunct to the Pap test only to screen for cervical cancer in women aged 30 years and older.

What Is the Relationship Between Cervical Cancer and HPV?

Infection with HPV is a necessary factor in the development of cervical cancer. More than 30 HPV types can infect the genital tract and are divided into 2 groups based on their association with cervical cancer.

- Low-risk types (such as 6 and 11, which cause 90% of genital warts)

- High-risk types (such as 16 and 18, which cause 70% of cervical cancers)

Most genital HPV infections are transient, asymptomatic, and have no clinical consequences. However, more than 99% of cervical cancers have HPV DNA detected within the tumor. The time from initial HPV infection to carcinoma in situ is 7 to 15 years.

Human papillomavirus is the most common sexually transmitted infection (STI) in the United States. At least one-half of sexually active individuals will be infected with HPV at some point in their lifetime. The HPV rates are highest in adolescents, with a cumulative incidence of up to 44% among 15- to 19-year-olds over 3 years and 60% at 5 years.

Risk factors for acquisition of HPV include, but are not limited to, multiple sex partners, younger age at sexarche, young age, and a sex partner with multiple partners.

Immunization can prevent HPV infection. Prophylactic HPV vaccines significantly reduces the rates of HPV infection and cervical cancer. Bivalent vaccines are used against types 16 and 18. Quadrivalent vaccines are used against types 6, 11, 16, and 18.

When Should You Screen for Cervical Dysplasia?

The American Cancer Society (2002)[1] recommends the first Pap test approximately 3 years after onset of vaginal intercourse, but no later than age 21. Screening should be done annually with conventional Pap test or liquid-based cytology until age 30. After age 30, Pap tests may be done every 2 to 3 years after 3 normal tests.

SCREENING

The US Preventive Services Task Force (USPSTF)[2] recommends the first Pap test within 3 years of onset of sexual activity or age 21, whichever comes first. Screening should be done at least every 3 years with conventional Pap test. The USPSTF found insufficient evidence for the use of liquid-based cytology.

The American College of Gynecology[3] recommends that cervical cancer screening begin at age 21 with either a conventional Pap test or liquid-based cytology regardless of the age of onset of sexual intercourse. Screening should be done every 2 years until age 30 and subsequently every 3 years after 3 consecutive normal tests. More frequent screening may be required for those who are immunosuppressed or infected with human immunodeficiency virus (HIV). Cervical cytology screening should be initiated in HIV-infected women at the time of diagnosis rather than deferring until age 21.

This new recommendation from ACOG was made because invasive cervical cancer is rare in women younger than age 21 (estimated incidence 1–2 cases per 1 million females aged 15–19). In addition, there has been overuse of follow-up procedures with an increase in premature births in women who previously had excisional biopsy for dysplasia.

How Should You Perform Cervical Dysplasia Screening?

Pap Test

Obtain a Pap test during a speculum examination with the cervix in full view, before STI tests, without lubricant, and preferably not during menses or in the presence of a known STI. The sample must include the squamocolumnar junction and the endocervix.

A Pap test can be performed using 1 of 2 methods: (1) the conventional method using slides or (2) liquid-based cytology. Instead of spreading cells onto a slide as in a conventional Pap test, in liquid-based cytology (Thinprep or SurePath), the cells are suspended in a preservative fluid. Liquid-based cytology can reduce cell overlap, obscuring blood, mucus, and inflammation. This test also allows for HPV DNA testing, although not recommended for adolescents.

Conventional Method: Spatula and Cytobrush

- Rotate a spatula with pressure around the cervix and spread the sample onto one slide.

- Insert a cytobrush into the cervical os and rotate gently. Roll the sample onto a second slide.

- As an alternative, both samples can be put on one slide per instructions from the laboratory.

- Fix the slides immediately with a spray fixative or place into a bottle of Pap fixative.

Conventional Method: Cervical Broom

- Rotate a cervical broom device with pressure around the cervix to collect both a cervical and endocervical sample simultaneously.

- Spread the collected material thinly on a slide.

- Fix the slides immediately with a spray fixative or place into a bottle of Pap fixative.

Liquid-Based Cytology: Spatula and Cytobrush Method

- Rotate a spatula with pressure around the cervix.

- Rotate a cytobrush gently in the cervical os.

- Vigorously swirl the spatula in the preservative medium and rub the cytobrush against the side of the collection vial to remove cells from the device.

Liquid-Based Cytology: Cervical Broom Method

- Rotate a cervical broom device with pressure around the cervix to collect both a cervical and endocervical sample simultaneously.

- Vigorously compress broom against the base of the collection vial 10 times to separate the cells from the device.

What Should You Do With an Abnormal Result?

If choosing to do a pap smear on an adolescent, guidelines from 2007, provide the following guidance for women ages 20 years and younger:

- For women with LSIL and aytpical squamous cells of undetermined significance (ASCUS), a repeat Pap is recommended in 12 months.

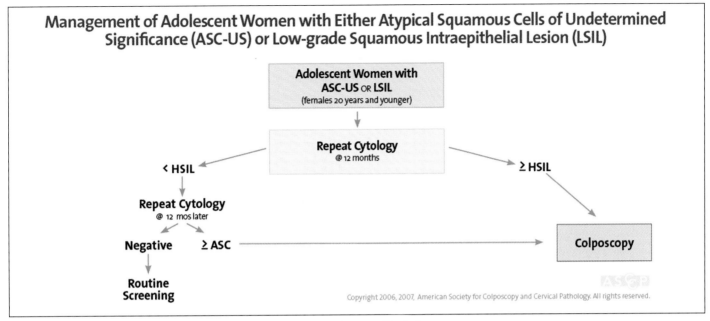

Management of Adolescent Women with Either Atypical Squamous Cells of Undetermined Significance (ASC-US) or Low-grade Squamous Intraepithelial Lesion (LSIL)

Used with permission from the American Society for Colposcopy and Cervical Pathology.

- At the 12-month follow-up, those with high-grade squamous intraepithelial lesions (HSIL) or greater should be referred for colposcopy.

- At the 24-month follow-up, those with ASCUS or greater should be referred for colposcopy.

Human papillomavirus DNA testing is not recommended for adolescents. If HPV testing is inadvertently performed, the results should not influence management. Colposcopy is not recommended for initial evaluation of LSIL or ASCUS cytology results in adolescents.

- All patients with atypical squamous cells that cannot be excluded as high-grade squamous intraepithelial lesions are referred directly for colposcopy.

- All patients with atypical glandular cells are referred directly for colposcopy.

- All patients with HSIL are referred directly for colposcopy.

What Results Should We Document?

Date of Pap test, Pap test results, recommendations for next Pap test, and referral for colposcopy.

ICD-9-CM Codes

795.01	Pap test with atypical squamous cells of undetermined significance (ASCUS)
795.02	Pap test with atypical squamous cells cannot exclude high-grade squamous intraepithelial lesion (ASC-H)
795.03	Pap test with low-grade squamous intraepithelial lesion (LGSIL)
795.04	Pap test with high-grade squamous intraepithelial lesion (HGSIL)
795.00	Pap test with atyupical glandular cells (AGC)

The American Academy of Pediatrics publishes a complete line of coding publications including an annual edition of *Coding for Pediatrics*. For more information on these excellent resources, visit the American Academy of Pediatrics online bookstore at **www.aap.org/bookstore/.**

Resources

Guidelines

American Society for Colposcopy and Cervical Pathology. *2006 Consensus Guidelines for the Management of Women with Abnormal Cervical Cancer Screening Tests.* American Society for Colposcopy and Cervical Pathology Web site. http://www.asccp.org/consensus/cytological.shtml

Institute for Clinical Systems Improvement. *2008 Revised Guidelines for Initial Management of Abnormal Cervical Cytology and HPV Testing.*

Articles

Baseman JG, Koutsky LA. The epidemiology of human papillomavirus. *J Clin Virol.* 2005:32S:S16–S24

Brown DR, Shew ML, Qadadri B, et al. A longitudinal study of genital human papillomavirus infection in a cohort of closely followed adolescent women. *J Infect Dis.* 2005;191:182–192

Cates W Jr. Estimates of the incidence and prevalence of sexually transmitted diseases in the United States. American Social Health Association Panel. *Sex Transm Dis.* 1999;26:S2–S7

Emans SJ, Laufer MR, Goldstein DP, eds. *Pediatric and Adolescent Gynecology.* 5th ed. Philadelphia, PA: Lippincott Williams & Wilkins; 2005

Guido R. Guidelines for screening and treatment of cervical disease in the adolescent. *J Pediatr Adolesc Gynecol.* 2004;17:303–311

Institute for Clinical Systems Improvement (ICSI). *Initial Management of Abnormal Cervical Cytology (Pap Smear) and HPV Testing.* Bloomington, MN: Institute for Clinical Systems Improvement; 2008

Kahn JA. Vaccination as a prevention strategy for human papillomavirus–related diseases. *J Adolesc Health.* 2005;37:S10–S16

Koutsky L. Epidemiology of genital human papillomavirus infection. *Am J Med.* 1997;102:3–8

Moscicki AB, Schiffman M, Kjaer S et al. Chapter 5: Updating the natural history of HPV and anogenital cancer. *Vaccine.* 2006;S3:S42–S51

Moscicki AB. Impact of HPV infection in adolescent populations. *J Adolesc Health.* 2005;37:S3–S9

Moscicki AB, Shiboski S, Hills NK, et al. Regression of low-grade squamous intra-epithelial lesions in young women. *Lancet.* 2004;364:1642–1644

Moscicki AB, Hills N, Shiboski S, et al. Risks for incident human papillomavirus infection and low-grade squamous intraepithelial lesion development in young females. *JAMA.* 2001;285:2995–3002

Munoz N, Bosch FX, de Sanjose S, et al. Epidemiologic classification of human papillomavirus type associated with cervical cancer. *N Engl J Med.* 2003;348:518–527

Neinstein LS, ed. *Adolescent Health Care: A Practical Guide.* 4th ed. Philadelphia, PA: Lippincott Williams & Wilkins; 2002

Schiffman M, Castle PE, Jeronimo J, et al. Human papillomavirus and cervical cancer. *Lancet.* 2007;370:890–907

Weinstock H, Berman S, Cates W Jr. Sexually transmitted diseases among American youth: incidence and prevalence estimates, 2000. *Perspect Sex Reprod Health.* 2004;36:6–10

Wright TC, Massad LS, Dunton CJ, et al. 2006 consensus guidelines for the management of women with abnormal cervical cancer screening tests. *Am J Obstet Gynecol.* 2007;197(4):346–355

Web Sites for Health Professionals

The American College of Obstetricians and Gynecologists: www.acog.org

American Cancer Society: www.cancer.org

CDC National Breast and Cervical Cancer Early Detection Program: http://www.cdc.gov/cancer/nbccedp/index.htm

US Preventive Services Task Force: www.ahrq.gov/clinic/uspstfix.htm

Web Sites for Adolescents and Parents

American Academy of Family Physicians: http://www.familydoctor.org/handouts/223.html

Center for Young Women's Health, Boston Children's Hospital: http://www.youngwomenshealth.org/abpap.html

National Women's Health Information Center, US Department of Health and Human Services: http://www.womenshealth.gov/faq/cervical-cancer.cfm

References

1. Watson, M, Saraiya M. Benard V et al. Burden of cervical cancer in the United States, 1998–2003, Cancer 2008:113:2855–2864.

2. American College of Obstetrics and Gynecology. ACOG practice bulletin. Number 109. Cervical cytology screening. Obstet Gynecol. 2009;114:1409–1420

3. U.S. Preventive Services Task Force. *Screening for Cervical Cancer: Recommendations and Rationale.* Rockville, MD: Agency for Healthcare Research and Quality; 2003. AHRQ Publication No. 03–515A. http://www.ahrq.gov/clinic/3rduspstf/cervcan/cervcanrr.htm

FRANCES PAGE GLASCOE, MD

DEVELOPMENTAL AND BEHAVIORAL CONSIDERATIONS

Developmental and behavioral surveillance and screening are recommended across the Bright Futures visits, with specific screening at various ages, including autism screening at the 18-month and 2-year visits and a structured developmental screen at the 9-month, 18-month, and 2½-year visits. Use of quality tools rather than informal methods, such as milestones checklists (even if drawn from longer screens), greatly improves detection rates. Rationale, policy, and useful accurate tools are described in this chapter.

Why Is It Important to Screen for Developmental and Behavioral Disabilities?

Screening confirms normal development and identifies developmental risks or disabilities.

Developmental disabilities are the most common disorders among children and adults, rivaling only asthma and obesity.[1,2] Studies indicate that 16% to 18% of all children aged 0 to 18 have developmental disabilities. In the 0 to 2-year age range alone, incidence reaches 13%.[1,2] Approximately 12% of school-aged children receive special education.

Healthy People 2010 identifies developmental disabilities as one of the 6 most important health concerns in the United States.

The most common disability (and also the least detected) is speech-language impairment, followed by learning disabilities and intellectual disabilities. Attention-deficit/hyperactivity disorder is the most common behavioral disorder. Less common (but somewhat more frequently detected) are autism, motor impairment, traumatic brain injury, and visual and hearing impairment.[3]

Poverty and other psychosocial risk factors are the leading cause of school failure and dropping out. Nationally, high school drop out rates average 20%. For inner-city, particularly minority youths, drop out rates often exceed 50% (www.uscensus.gov). Such at-risk children not only have psychosocial challenges but also deficits in skills essential to school success: language, academics, and cognition.[4,5]

Developmental and behavioral screening is recommended. The National Guideline Clearinghouse concludes there is good evidence to recommend screening for a range of conditions.

An American Academy of Pediatrics (AAP) policy statement urges clinicians to screen for developmental-behavioral problems at health supervision visits using quality tools.[6]

The AAP also encourages routine developmental-behavioral surveillance during health supervision visits (see the "Developmental Strengths" chapter). Surveillance provides "the big picture" of children's and families' needs and encompasses

- Viewing and addressing psychosocial risk factors and parents' concerns

- Monitoring developmental and behavioral progress

- Promoting resilience (eg, positive parenting practices) through parent education

- Referring to a wide range of programs (eg, quality day care, parent training classes, social services, etc)[6]

Disabilities can be ameliorated through early intervention and sometimes prevented. Early intervention (EI) takes many forms. Whether through Head Start, Early Head Start, quality day care, or public school services, EI programs lead to dramatically improved outcomes. These include decreases in teen pregnancy, high school dropout, criminality, unemployment, and secondary emotional problems.[4]

Both surveillance and screening can be readily accomplished during health supervision visits. Use of evidence-based tools for both tasks (often one and the same) contain, if not reduce, visit length. It also increases the likelihood of families returning for well visits, improves parent and clinician satisfaction with care, and enhances reimbursement.[7–10]

When and With Whom Should You Perform a Developmental-Behavioral Screen?

Only 25% of those eligible for EI are detected and enrolled.[11] Prevention and intervention depend on the use of accurate screening tools and actions to ensure that the results are used to direct families to needed referral resources.[4,11–14] Informal techniques, such as milestones checklists (even when they are drawn from larger measures), detect fewer than 30% of all children with developmental disabilities—and thus only the more severe cases.[7,11,15]

Routine feedback to health care providers on the accuracy of their early detection methods is lacking. Deploying quality improvement techniques (now a required part of residency training) is helpful. At a minimum, view your referral rates in light of prevalence: About 1 out of every 6 children needs some form of developmental or behavioral intervention.[1,2,11]

Whom to Screen

- Administer screening tests to **asymptomatic** children.

When to Screen

- 9-month visit

- 18-month visit

- 2-year visit (if a 2½-year visit will not be completed)

- 2½-year visit

Following the 2½-year visit, administer a validated, standardized, and accurate screening test at all annual health supervision visits based on developmental surveillance and clinical judgment. The tests should be broad in scope, meaning that they sample all developmental domains.

- At the 18-month and 2-year visits, add an autism spectrum disorder (ASD)-specific tool.

Screens that use only ASD-specific tools will miss most children with other conditions. Therefore, use an ASD screen only in conjunction with a broad-band screen and never as the sole measure of development and behavior.

The AAP policy statement, "Identifying Infants and Young Children With Developmental Disorders in the Medical Home: An Algorithm for Developmental Surveillance and Screening," also recommends screening all children for whom a developmental concern is raised by the parent or pediatrician. In addition, the statement recommends health care practitioners should perform developmental surveillance or formal developmental screening to evaluate a child's readiness for kindergarten at the 4- or 5-year-old health supervision visit.

What to Do

- At every health supervision visit, provide developmental surveillance.

  - Elicit and respond to parents' concerns.

  - Observe child and parent behavior.

  - Review medical history and current health status.

  - Monitor milestones.

  - Promote development through patient education.

  - Periodically screen for parental depression (see "Maternal Depression" chapter).

  - Assess psychosocial risk factors.

- At the visits noted above, administer accurate screening tools. Some tools also provide evidence-based approaches to surveillance. See the Resources section for a table listing evidence-based screening and surveillance measures.

What Should You Do With an Abnormal Result?

When children fail specific screening items or if surveillance activities suggest the presence of a problem, make a prompt referral to either EI services or, **for children 3 and older,** to public school special education. Either agency will provide additional evaluations without charge to families.

A diagnosis is not required by EI services. Only a percentage of delay (eg, 1.5 standard deviations or 40% below chronological age in one developmental domain) is needed to establish eligibility. Criteria vary somewhat by state.

Referrals to private diagnostic services also can be made, but it is inadvisable to delay intervention while children wait for additional evaluations (eg, from an autism specialist). Developmental disabilities are best treated even before the diagnosis is final, particularly in children 5 and younger.

Early intervention and public school programs often require vision and hearing screening before they can evaluate referred children. Where possible, administer such screens (and also lead screening), and document results along with recommendations for the types of evaluations most needed (eg, audiological, speech-language).

It is important to recognize that early intervention can take many forms. When children do not qualify for special services, refer for other forms of intervention such as Head Start, quality day care, and/or parenting classes.

What Results and Referrals Should You Document?

Documentation

- Unbundle procedure code *(CPT)* 96110 (developmental screening) from the health supervision visit code (typically with modifier 25) and bill separately (2004 Medicaid ruling). Many private payers, as of publication, reimburse 96110 separately. The 2010 Medicare Fee Schedule (non-facility) for 96110 is $7.21, and payments from private payers may be more or less depending on the negotiated fee schedule.

- When screening results are problematic, use general diagnosis codes so as not to interfere with codes used in subsequent evaluations (see examples of general codes in the *ICD-9-CM* codes section).

Referrals

- Most EI programs have a referral form that you can use to document results. Request these forms directly from programs.

- A brief referral letter is sufficient, but it is helpful to suggest the types of evaluations needed (most particularly speech-language). Also document results of hearing and vision screens in your referral letter.

- If possible, establish a 2-way consent process so that parents agree that the referral resource can share results of additional testing with health care providers.

- For locating services for school-aged children, call the school psychologist or speech-language pathologist in the child's school of zone.

ICD-9-CM Codes	
783.42	Delayed milestones
315.8	Other specific delays in development
315.9	Unspecified delays in development
348.30	Unspecified encephalopathy
348.9	Unspecified condition of brain
315.9	Unspecified delays in development (including academic delays)
781.3	Lack of coordination (eg, hypotonia, hypertonia, incoordination)
781.9	Abnormalities of the muscle, skeletal, or nervous system

The American Academy of Pediatrics publishes a complete line of coding publications, including an annual edition of *Coding for Pediatrics*. For more information on these excellent resources, visit the American Academy of Pediatrics Online Bookstore at **www.aap.org/bookstore/**.

Resources

Articles

Sices L, Feudtner C, McLaughlin J, Drotar D, Williams M. How do primary care physicians manage children with possible developmental delays? A national survey with experimental design. *Pediatrics.* 2004;113:274–282

Silverstein M, Sand N, Glascoe FP, Gupta B, Tonniges T, O'Conner K. Pediatricians' reported practices regarding developmental screening: do guidelines work? Do they help? *Pediatrics.* 2005;116:174–179

Tools for Screening and Surveillance

The following table lists of measures that meet standards for screening test accuracy, meaning that they correctly identify, at all ages, at least 70% of children with disabilities while also correctly identifying at least 70%

children without disabilities. All included measures were standardized on national samples, proven to be reliable, and validated against a range of measures.

The first column provides publication information and the cost of purchasing a specimen set. The "Description" column provides information on alternative ways, if available, to administer measures (eg, waiting rooms). The "Accuracy" column shows the percentage of patients with and without problems identified correctly. The "Time Frame/Costs" column shows the costs of materials per visit along with the costs of professional time (using the an average salary of $50 per hour) needed to administer and interpret each measure. Time/cost estimates do not include expenses associated with referring. For parent report tools, administration time reflects not only scoring of test results, but also the relationship between each test's reading level and the percentage of parents with less than a high school education (who may or may

Evidence-based Screening and Surveillance Measures

BEHAVIORAL and/or DEVELOPMENTAL SCREENS RELYING ON INFORMATION FROM PARENTS	Age Range	Description	Scoring	Accuracy	Time Frame/ Costs
Parents' Evaluations of Developmental Status (PEDS). (2002) Ellsworth & Vandermeer Press, Ltd. 1013 Austin Court, Nolensville, TN 37135 Phone: 615-776-4121; fax: 615-776-4119 http://www.pedstest.com ($36.00) PEDS is also available online together with the Modified Checklist of Autism in Toddlers for electronic records.	Birth to 8 years	10 questions eliciting parents' concerns with decision-guidance for providers. In English, Spanish , Vietnamese and many other languages. Written at the 4th–5th grade level. Determines when to refer, provide a second screen, provide patient education, or monitor development, behavior/emotional, and academic progress. Provides longitudinal surveillance and triage	Identifies children as low, moderate or high risk for various kinds of disabilities and delays	Sensitivity ranging from 74% to 79% and specificity ranging from 70% to 80% across age levels.	About 2 minutes (if interview needed) Print Materials ~$.39 $1.20 Total = ~$1.59
Ages and Stages Questionnaire-3 (formerly Infant Monitoring System) (2004). Paul H. Brookes Publishing, Inc., PO Box 10624, Baltimore, MD 21285 (1-800-638-3775). ($199.95) http://www.pbrookes.com/	4 to 60 months	Parents indicate children's developmental skills on 25–35 items (4 – 5 pages) using a different form for each well visit. Reading level varies across items from 3rd to 12th grade. Can be used in mass mail-outs for child-find programs. In English, Spanish, French	Pass/fail and monitor score for developmental status	Sensitivity ranged 70% to 90% at all ages except the 4 month level. Specificity ranged from 76% to 91%	about 15 minutes (if interview needed) Materials ~$.40 Admin. ~$2.40 Total = ~$2.80

BEHAVIORAL and/or DEVELOPMENTAL SCREENS RELYING ON INFORMATION FROM PARENTS (continued)	Age Range	Description	Scoring	Accuracy	Time Frame/ Costs
Infant-Toddler Checklist for Language and Communication (1998). Paul H. Brookes Publishing, Inc., P.O. Box 10624, Baltimore, MD, 21285 (1-800-638-3775). (Part of CSBS-DP, $ http://www.pbrookes.com/ ($99.95 w/ CD-ROM)	6–24 months	Parents complete the Checklist's 24 multiple-choice questions in English. Reading level is 6th grade. Based on screening for delays in language development as the first evident symptom that a child is not developing typically. Does not screen for motor milestones. The Checklist is copyrighted but remains free for use at the Brookes Web site although the factor scoring system is complicated and requires purchase of the CD-ROM.	Manual table of cut-off scores at 1.25 standard deviations below the mean OR an optional scoring CD-ROMs	Sensitivity is 78%; Specificity is 84%.	About 5 to 10 minutes Materials ~.$.20 Admin. ~$3.40 Total ~$3.60
PEDS- Developmental Milestones (PEDS-DM (2007) Online at: PEDSTest.comLLC 1013 Austin Court, Nolensville, TN 37135 Phone: 615-776-4121; fax: 615-776-4119 Online at: http://www.pedstest.com ($275.00)	0–8 years	PEDS-DM consists of 6–8 items at each age level (spanning the well visit schedule). Each item taps a different domain (fine/gross motor, self-help, academics, expressive/receptive language, social-emotional). Items are administered by parents or professionals. Forms are laminated and marked with a grease pencil. It can be used to complement PEDS or stand alone. Administered by parent report or directly. Written at the 2nd grade level. A longitudinal score form tracks performance. Supplemental measures also included include the M-CHAT, Family Psychosocial Screen, PSC-17, the SWILS, the Vanderbilt, and a measure of parent-child interactions. An Assessment Level version is available for NICU follow-up and early intervention programs. In English and Spanish.	Cutoffs tied to performance above and below the 16th percentile for each item and its domain. On the Assessment equivalent scores are produced and enable users to compute percentage of delays.	Sensitivity (.75–.87); specificity (.71–.88 to performance in each domain. Sensitivity (.70–.94); specificity (.77–.93) across age	About 3–5 Materials ~.$.02 Admin. ~$1.00 Total ~$1.02

BEHAVIORAL/EMOTIONAL SCREENS RELYING ON INFORMATION FROM PARENTS	Age Range	Description	Scoring	Accuracy	Time Frame/ Costs
Eyberg Child Behavior Inventory/ Sutter-Eyberg Student Behavior Inventory. Psychological Assessment Resources, P.O. Box 998 Odessa Florida: 33556 (1-800-331-8378) ($120.00) http://www.parinc.com/	2 to 16 years of age	The ECBI/SESBI consists of 36–38 short statements of common behavior problems. More than 16 suggests the referrals for behavioral interventions. Fewer than 16 enables the measure to function as a problems list for planning in-office counseling, selecting handouts, and monitoring progress.	Single refer/nonrefer score for externalizing problems,— conduct, aggression, etc.	Sensitivity 80%, specificity 86% to disruptive behavior problems	About 7 minutes (if interview needed) Materials ~$.30 Admin. ~$2.38 Total = ~$2.68
Pediatric Symptom Checklist. Jellinek MS, Murphy JM, Robinson J, et al. Pediatric Symptom Checklist: Screening school age children for academic and psychosocial dysfunction. http://psc.partners.org/ The Pictorial PSC, useful with low-income Spanish speaking families can be downloaded freely at www.dbpeds.org (included in the PEDS:DM)	4–16 years.	35 short statements of problem behaviors including both externalizing (conduct) and internalizing (depression, anxiety, adjustment, etc.) Ratings of never, sometimes or often are assigned a value of 0,1,or 2. Scores totaling 28 or more suggest referrals. Factor scores identify attentional, internalizing and externalizing problems. Factor scoring is available for download at: http://www.pedstest.com/links/resources.html	Single refer/nonrefer score	All but one study showed high sensitivity (80% to 95%) but somewhat scattered specificity (68%–100%).	About 7 minutes (if interview needed) Materials ~$.10 Admin. ~$2.38 Total = ~$2.48
Parents' Evaluations of Developmental Status (PEDS). (2002) Ellsworth & Vandermeer Press, Ltd. 1013 Austin Court, Nolensville, TN 37135 Phone: 615-776-4121; fax: 615-776-4119 http://www.pedstest.com ($36.00) PEDS is also available online together with the Modified Checklist of Autism in Toddlers for electronic records.	Birth to 8 years	10 questions eliciting parents' concerns in English, Spanish , Vietnamese and many other languages. Written at the 4th - 5th grade level. Determines when to refer, provide a second screen, provide patient education, or monitor development, behavior/ emotional, and academic progress. Provides longitudinal surveillance and triage.	Identifies children as low, moderate or high risk for various kinds of disabilities and delays	Sensitivity ranging from 74% to 79% and specificity ranging from 70% to 80% across age levels.	About 2 minutes (if interview needed) Print Materials ~$.39 Admin. ~$1.20 Total = ~$1.59

BEHAVIORAL/EMOTIONAL SCREENS RELYING ON INFORMATION FROM PARENTS	Age Range	Description	Scoring	Accuracy	Time Frame/ Costs
Ages & Stages Questionnaires: Social-Emotional (ASQ:SE) Paul H. Brookes, Publishers, PO Box 10624, Baltimore, Maryland 21285 (1-800-638-3775). ($125) http://www.pbrookes.com/	6–60 months	Designed to supplement the ASQ, the ASQ SE consists of 30 item forms (4–5 pages long) for each of 8 visits between 6 and 60 months. Items focus on self-regulation, compliance, communication, adaptive functioning, autonomy, affect, and interaction with people	Single cutoff score indicating when a referral is needed	Sensitivity ranged from 71%–85%. Specificity from 90% to 98%	10–15 minutes if interview needed. Materials ~ $.40 ~$4.20 Total = ~ $4.40
Brief-Infant-Toddler Social-Emotional Assessment (BITSEA); Harcourt Assessment, Inc, 19500 Bulverde Road	San Antonio, Texas 78259 |(1-800-211-8378) ($99.00) harcourtassessment.com	12–36 months	42 item parent-report measure for identifying social-emotional/ behavioral. problems and delays in competence. Items were drawn from the assessment level measure, the ITSEA. Written at the 4th–6th grade level. Available in Spanish, French, Dutch, Hebrew	Cut-points based on child age and sex show present/ absence of problems and competence.	Sensitivity (80–85%) in detecting children with social-emotional/ behavioral problems and specificity 75% to 80%.	5–7 minutes Materials ~$1.15 Admin. ~$.88 Total ~$2.03
PEDS- Developmental Milestones (PEDS-DM (2007) PEDSTest.comLLC P.O. Box 68164 Nashville, Tennessee 37206 Phone: 615-226-4460; fax: 615-227-0411 ($275.00) Online at: http://www.pedstest.com	0–8 years	PEDS-DM consists of 6–8 items at each age level (spanning the well visit schedule). Each item taps a different domain (fine/ gross motor, self-help, academics, expressive/ receptive language, social-emotional). Items are administered by parents or professionals. Forms are laminated and marked with a grease pencil. It can be used to complement PEDS or stand alone. Administered by parent report or directly. Written at the 2nd grade level. A longitudinal score form tracks performance. Supplemental measures also included include the M-CHAT, Family Psychosocial Screen, PSC-17, the SWILS, the VAnderbilt, and a measure of parent-child interactions. An Assessment Level version is available for NICU follow-up and early intervention programs. In English and Spanish.	Cutoffs tied to performance above and below the 16th percentile for each item and its domain. On the Assessment Level, age equivalent scores are produced and enable users to compute percentage of delays.	Sensitivity (.75–.87); specificity (.71–.88 to performance in each domain. Sensitivity (.70–.94); specificity (.77 - .93) across age	About 3–5 minutes Materials ~.$.02 Admin. ~$1.00 Total ~$1.02

FAMILY SCREENS	Age Range	Description	Scoring	Accuracy	Time Frame/ Costs
Family Psychosocial Screening. Kemper, KJ & Kelleher KJ. Family psychosocial screening: instruments and techniques. Ambulatory Child Health. 1996;4:325-339. (the measures are included in the article) and downloadable at http://www.pedstest.com (included in the PEDS:DM)	screens parents and best used along with the above screens	A two-page clinic intake form that identifies psychosocial risk factors associated with developmental problems including: a four item measure of parental history of physical abuse as a child; (2) a six item measure of parental substance abuse;and (3) a three item measure of maternal depression.	Refer/nonrefer scores for each risk factor. Also has guides to referring and resource lists.	All studies showed sensitivity and specificity to larger inventories greater than 90%	about 15 minutes (if interview needed) Materials ~$.20 Admin. ~$4.20 Total = ~$4.40

DEVELOPMENTAL SCREENS RELYING ON ELICITING SKILLS DIRECTLY FROM CHILDREN

	Age Range	Description	Scoring	Accuracy	Time Frame/ Costs
Brigance Screens-II. Curriculum Associates, Inc. (2005) 153 Rangeway Road, N. Billerica, MA, 01862 (1-800-225-0248 ($501.00). http://www.curriculumassociates.com/	0–90 months	Nine separate forms, one for each 12 month age range. Taps speech-language, motor, readiness and general knowledge at younger ages and also reading and math at older ages. Uses direct elicitation and observation. In the 0–2 administered by parent report	Cutoff, quotients, percentiles, age equivalent scores in various domains and overall.	Sensitivity and specificity to giftedness and to develop-mental and academic problems are 70% to 82% across ages	10–15 minutes Materials ~$1.53 Admin. ~$10.15 Total = ~$11.68
Bayley Infant Neurodevelomental Screen (BINS). San Antonio, Texas: The Psychological Corporation, 1995. 555 Academic Court, San Antonio, TX 78204 (1-800-228-0752) ($265) http://www.psychcorp.com	3–24 months	Uses 10–13 directly elicited items per 3–6 month age range assess neurological processes (reflexes, and tone); neurodevelopmental skills (movement, and symmetry) and developmental accomplishments (object permanence, imitation, and language).	Categorizes performance into low, moderate or high risk via cut scores. Provides subtest cut scores for each domain	Specificity and sensitivity are 75% to 86% across ages	10–15 minutes Materials ~$.30 Admin. ~$10.15 Total = ~$10.45
Battelle Developmental Inventory Screening Test–II (BDIST)–2 (2006). Riverside Publishing Company, 8420 Bryn Mawr Avenue, Chicago, Illinois 60631 (1-800-323-9540) ($239 www.riversidepublishing.com	0–95 months	Items (20 per domain) use a combination of direct assessment, observation, and parental interview. A high level of examiner skill is required. Well standardized and validated. Scoring software including a PDA application is available. English and Spanish	Age equivalents and cutoffs at 1.0, 1.5, and 2.0 SDs below the mean in each of 5 domains	Sensitivity (72% to 93%) to various disabilities; Specificity (79% to 88%). Accuracy information across age ranges is not available.	10–30 minutes Materials ~$1.65 Admin. ~$20.15 Total = ~$21.80

ACADEMIC SCREENS	Age Range	Description	Scoring	Accuracy	Time Frame/ Costs
Comprehensive Inventory of Basic Skills-Revised Screener (CIBS-R Screener) Curriculum Associates, Inc. (1985) 153 Rangeway Road, N. Billerica, MA, 01862 (1-800-225-0248 ($224.00). http://www.curriculum associates.com/	1–6th grade	Administration involves one or more of three subtests (reading comprehension, math computation, and sentence writing). Timing performance also enables an assessment of information processing skills, especially rate.	Computerized or hand-scoring produces percentiles, quotients, cutoffs	70% to 80% accuracy across all grades	Takes 10–15 minutes Materials ~$.53 Admin. ~$10.15 Total = ~$10.68
Safety Word Inventory and Literacy Screener (SWILS). Glascoe FP, Clinical Pediatrics, 2002. Items courtesy of Curriculum Associates, Inc. The SWILS can be freely downloaded at: http://www. pedstest.com/	6–14	Children are asked to read 29 common safety words (e.g., High Voltage, Wait, Poison) aloud. The number of correctly read words is compared to a cutoff score. Results predict performance in math, written language and a range of reading skills. Test content may serve as a springboard to injury prevention counseling.	single cutoff score indicating the need for a referral	78% to 84% sensitivity and specificity across all ages	about 7 minutes (if interview needed) Materials ~$.30 Admin. ~$2.38 Total = ~$2.68
Narrow-Band Screens for AUTISM and ADHD					
Modified Checklist for Autism in Toddlers (M-CHAT) (1997). Free download at the First Signs Web site: http://www.firstsigns.org/downloads /m-chat.PDF ($0.00) Online for parents and EMRS at www.forepath.org ($1.00) (also included in the PEDS:DM)	18–60 months	Parent report of 23 questions modified for American usage at 4–6th grade reading level. Available in English and Spanish. Uses telephone follow-up for concerns. The M-CHAT is copyrighted but remains free for use on the First Signs Web site. The full text article appeared in the April 2001 issue of the *Journal of Autism and Developmental Disorders*.	Cutoff based on 2 of 3 critical items or any 3 from checklist.	Initial study shows sensitivity at 90%; specificity at 99%. Future studies are needed for a full picture. Promising tool.	About 5 minutes Print Materials ~$.10 Admin. ~$.88 Total = ~$.98
Conners Rating Scales-Revised (CRS-R) Multi-Health Systems, Inc. P.O. Box 950, North Tonawanda, NY 14120-0950 Call 1.800.456.3003 or +1.416.492.2627 Fax 1.888.540.4484 or 1.416.492.3343 http://www.mhs.com/ ($193.00)	3 to 17 years	Although the CRSR can screen for a range of problems, Several subscales specific to ADHD are included: DSM-IV symptom subscales (Inattentive, Hyperactive/Impulsive, and Total); Global Indices (Restless-Impulsive, Emotional Lability, and Total), and an ADHD Index. The GI is useful for treatment monitoring. Also available in French	Cutoff tied to the 93rd percentile for each factor	Sensitivity 78% to 92% Specificity: 84% to 94%	About 20 minutes Materials ~$.2.25 Admin. ~$20.15 Total = ~$22.40

not be able to complete measures in waiting rooms due to literacy problems and thus will need interview administrations).

Please note: Not included are measures such as the Denver-II that fail to meet standards (limited standardization, absent validation, and no proof of accuracy) or measures of single developmental domains (eg, just language or motor).

Web Sites

Administration for Children and Families: www.acf.hhs.gov
To locate social services addressing domestic violence, housing and food instability, child abuse and neglect, adoption, state, and local services, etc.

American Academy of Pediatrics: http://www.aap.org/
Identifying infants and young children with developmental disorders in the medical home: an algorithm for developmental surveillance and screening (2006).

American Academy of Pediatrics Medical Home: http://www.medicalhomeinfo.org/tools/coding.html
Web site with information on coding, reimbursement, and advocacy assistance with denied claims. The broader Web site provides guidance on establishing a medical home for children with special needs.

American Academy of Pediatrics Section on Developmental and Behavioral Pediatrics: http://www.dbpeds.org
Provides information on screening, rationale, implementation, etc.

Bright Futures: http://www.brightfutures.app.org/
Guidelines and information on providing comprehensive health supervision services, case-based learning examples, etc.

Centers for Disease Control and Prevention: Developmental Screening to Improve Child Health: http://www.cdc.gov/ncbddd/child/improve.htm
Offers information on the value of screening with links to research and services, wall charts on milestones (helpful for alerting parents to health care providers' interest in child development).

Child Care Aware: www.childcareaware.org
To find quality preschool and day care programs.

Developmental Screening Tool Kit: www.developmentalscreening.org
Implementation guidance and research, with an excellent video of pediatricians and a hospital administrator at Harvard University showing opinions about screening before and after implementing a quality tool.

Early Head Start National Resource Center: www.ehsnrc.org
For help locating Head Start and Early Head Start programs.

First Signs: www.firstsigns.org
To find services and information about autism spectrum disorders.

Healthy People 2010: http://www.healthypeople.gov/Document/HTML/Volume1/06Disability.htm
Healthy People 2010 Chapter Six Disability and Secondary Conditions. Provides information on the initiative, goals, interventions, etc.

KidsHealth: www.kidshealth.org
For downloadable parenting information.

National Association for the Education of Young Children: www.naeyc.org/
To find quality preschool and day care programs.

National Early Childhood Technical Assistance Center: http://www.nectac.org
Provides links to early intervention and public school services in each state, region, and community.

National Guideline Clearinghouse: http://www.guideline.gov
Provides information on screening for many specific conditions including the American Academy of Neurology autism screening guidelines.

Parents as Teachers: www.patnc.org
For information on parent training programs.

Parents' Evaluation of Developmental Status: www.pedstest.com
Slide shows and other materials for teaching screening measures, a trial of online developmental-behavioral and autism screens, parent education handouts, and an early detection discussion list.

Substance Abuse and Mental Health Services' Administration National Mental Health Information Center: www.mentalhealth.org
For help locating mental health services

YWCA: www.ywca.org
For information on parent training programs.

References

1. Newacheck PW, Strickland B, Shonkoff JP. An epidemiologic profile of children with special health care needs. *Pediatrics*. 1998;102:117–123

2. Rosenberg SA, Zhang D, Robinson CC. Services for young children: prevalence of developmental delays and participation in early intervention. *Pediatrics*. 2008;121:e1503–e1509

3. Prelock PA, Hutchings T, Glascoe FP. Speech-language impairment: how to identify the most common and least diagnosed disability of childhood. *Medscape J Med*. 2008;10:136

4. Reynolds AJ, Temple JA, Ou S-R, Robertson DL, et al. Effects of a school-based, early childhood intervention on adult health and well-being: a 19-year follow-up of low-income families. *Arch Pediatr Adolesc Med*. 2007;161:730–739

5. Glascoe FP. Are over-referrals on developmental screening tests really a problem? *Arch Pediatr Adolesc Med*. 2001;155:54–59

6. American Academy of Pediatrics Council on Children With Disabilities, Section on Developmental Behavioral Pediatrics, Bright Futures Steering Committee, Medical Home Initiatives for Children With Special Needs Project Advisory Committee. Identifying infants and young children with developmental disorders in the medical home: an algorithm for developmental surveillance and screening. *Pediatrics*. 2006;118:405–420

7. Pappas D, Schonwald A. Developmental screening in primary care: a short overview of the process, challenges, and benefits of implementing a screening program. *AAP Developmental-Behavioral Pediatrics News*. October 2008

8. Magar NA, Dabova-Missova S, Gjerdingen DK. Effectiveness of targeted anticipatory guidance during well-child visits: a pilot trial. *J Am Board Fam Med*. 2006;19:450–458

9. Blair M, Hall D. From health surveillance to health promotion: the changing focus in preventive children's services. *Arch Dis Child*. 2006;91:730–735

10. Smith PK. Enhancing child development services in Medicaid managed care: a BCAP toolkit. Center for Health Care Strategies, Inc Web Site. 2005. http://www.chcs.org/usr_doc/Toolkit.pdf

11. Pinto-Martin JA, Dunkle M, Earls M, Fliedner D, Landes C. Developmental stages of developmental screening: steps to implementation of a successful program. *Am J Public Health*. 2005;95:1928–1932

12. Reynolds AJ, Temple JA, Robertson DL, Mann EA. Long-term effects of an early childhood intervention on educational achievement and juvenile arrest: a 15-year follow-up of low-income children in public schools. *JAMA*. 2001;285:2339–2346

13. Bailey DB, Hebbeler K, Scarborough A, Spiker D, Mallik S. First experiences with early intervention: a national perspective. *Pediatrics*. 2004;114:887–896

14. Bailey DB Jr, Skinner D, Warren SF. Newborn screening for developmental disabilities: reframing presumptive benefit. *Am J Public Health*. 2005;95:1889–1893

15. Hix-Small H, Marks K, Squires J, Nickel R. Impact of implementing developmental screening at 12 and 24 months in a pediatric practice. *Pediatrics*. 2007;120:381–389

ANN CLOCK EDDINS, PhD, CCC-A

HEARING

Although newborn universal screening captures much of congenital hearing loss, acquired hearing loss can manifest itself in childhood and be unrecognizable to the families or others. Thus hearing screening during childhood is recommended selectively based on risk assessment, and universally at designated preschool and school-age visits.

What Is Hearing Loss?

There are several types of hearing loss.

- **Conductive** hearing loss results from problems occurring in the outer and/or middle ears. On the audiogram, bone conduction thresholds are better than air conduction thresholds. This type of loss attenuates sound as it travels from the outer ear to the inner ear.

  Conductive loss is commonly caused by wax in the ear canal, fluid in the middle ear, or a tear in the eardrum, each of which can be treated medically or surgically. Depending on the cause of the loss, the child may experience pain and discomfort, prompting a caregiver to have the child's hearing tested. Less commonly occurring is conductive loss as a result of a congenital syndrome.

- **Sensorineural** hearing loss results from pathology associated with the inner ear and/or auditory nerve. On the audiogram, air conduction and bone conduction thresholds should be essentially the same within each ear, but can sometimes vary across the 2 ears depending on the underlying pathology. This type of loss can attenuate sound as well as distort sounds and speech to some degree.

  Common causes of sensorineural hearing loss in children include congenital factors (genetic, prenatal, perinatal, or postnatal infections) or acquired factors (ie, meningitis, ototoxicity associated with certain drugs).

- **Mixed** hearing loss is diagnosed when a child with sensorineural hearing loss also develops a conductive loss as a result of outer and/or middle ear pathologies. If the conductive hearing loss can be treated, the child may still have a sensorineural hearing loss. In a small portion of children, mixed hearing loss can be permanent and is associated with a congenital syndrome.

- **Central** hearing loss is the result of damage or dysfunction in the central auditory nervous system. This type of loss is due to space-occupying lesions (ie, brain tumors) and perceptual processing difficulties. Auditory neuropathy spectrum disorder is a dysfunction of the synapse of the inner hair cells and auditory nerve, and/or the auditory nerve itself.

Why Is It Important to Screen for Hearing Loss?

Hearing loss is the number one birth defect in the United States. In the United States, nearly 33 babies are born every day with permanent hearing loss and 1 in 1,000 have a profound hearing loss. Another 2 to 3 in 1,000 have partial hearing loss.

Screening based on risk identifies only a small portion of babies with hearing loss. For decades, screening for hearing loss in newborns was only done on those infants who were believed to be at high risk of hearing loss (eg, family history, low birth weight, hyperbilirubinemia, or external ear or facial deformities) or for infants in the neonatal intensive care unit.

SCREENING

However, nearly half of babies born with hearing loss do not exhibit an apparent risk factor. Therefore, risk-based screening programs identified fewer than 20% of infants with hearing loss.

The implementation of universal hearing screening programs has been successful in getting more than 95% of all newborns screened for hearing loss before being discharged from the hospital. Yet not all who fail the screening return for follow-up testing, and not all of those identified with a loss receive appropriate and timely follow-up services.

Delayed identification can affect language development and academic achievement. Studies show that infants and preschoolers with even a mild or unilateral hearing loss are at risk for language and other developmental delays, while school children with similar mild or unilateral losses are at risk for academic, social, and behavioral difficulties.[1-5] As many as 10% to 15% of school-aged children have some degree of hearing loss that affects their language development and learning.

In the past, most children with severe-profound hearing loss but no risk factors were not identified until an average age of 30 months. This is later than the critical period for optimal language development.[6-8]

Children with mild and moderate hearing loss or unilateral hearing loss were typically not identified until they enrolled in school.

Some forms of hearing loss develop after the newborn period. Although newborn hearing screening programs aim to identify newborns with congenital hearing loss, some forms of congenital hearing loss may not become evident until later in childhood. Similarly, hearing impairment can be acquired during infancy and childhood.

Infectious diseases, such as meningitis and otitis media, are two of the leading causes of acquired hearing loss in children.

Be ready to recognize children who may be at risk of late-developing congenital hearing loss or acquired hearing loss. Be prepared to evaluate hearing in these children or refer to hearing professionals (eg, otolaryngologist or audiologist) for evaluation and treatment.

If hearing loss is not detected by 6 months of age, there is an increased risk of delayed speech and language development; poor social, emotional, and cognitive development; and poorer academic development.[3,9,10]

Otitis media with effusion is associated with hearing loss. Otitis media with effusion (OME) can result in a mild to moderate conductive hearing loss, which can lead to a delay in speech and language development. Chronic OME is associated with poorer processing of complex auditory sounds in later childhood.[11,12]

More than 2 million cases of OME are diagnosed annually in the United States, with estimated direct and indirect costs of $4 billion.

Of children with OME, 90% present before school age and 30% to 40% have recurrent episodes. Of children with recurrent episodes, 5% to 10% of the episodes last 1 year or more.[13,14]

Hearing screening is often a covered service. Because state laws mandate newborn hearing screening, parents are not responsible for paying for the test. Diagnostic audiologic procedures beyond the initial newborn hearing screening are covered by Medicare, Medicaid, and most private health insurance plans and will pay for the hearing screen. Some private carriers may inappropriately bundle the hearing screen (*CPT* code **92551**) with the office visit. Hearing aids for infants and children, if needed, are generally covered by state or locally funded agencies and, depending on the health plan, by private carriers.

How Should You Screen for Hearing Loss?

Screening for Hearing Loss in Infants

Key benchmarks of the newborn and infant hearing screening process

- Perform a hearing screen no later than age 1 month.

- For infants who do not pass the screening, conduct a diagnostic audiologic evaluation no later than age 3 months.

- For those identified with hearing loss, enroll the infants in an early intervention program no later than age 6 months.

Figure 1.

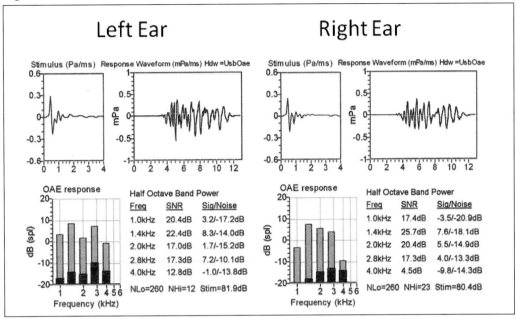

Source: Ann Clock Eddins, PhD, CCC-A

Types of procedures

Two types of electrophysiologic procedures are used, either alone or in combination, to screen newborns.

● **Otoacoustic emissions (OAE)** are soft sounds produced by most normal inner ears that cannot be heard by other people but can be recorded by sensitive microphones.

Otoacoustic emissions testing is painless and can be completed in about 5 minutes in a sleeping infant.

▷ Place a small soft probe tip in the ear canal. Present a series of clicks or tones through the probe and record the OAE response.

▷ Measure 2 common types of emissions: transient-evoked OAE (TEOAE) and distortion-product OAE.

Both types provide information about the functional status of outer hair cells (OHCs) in the inner ear over a range of frequencies important for speech processing and perception.

The OAEs are not a test of "hearing" per se, but they are a measure of OHC integrity and are typically present in individuals with normal hearing to a mild hearing loss (30–40 decibel level [dB HL] [hearing level in decibels]).

Figure 1 shows an example of a normal TEOAE. A passed screening is determined by the signal-to-noise ratio (SNR) in dB (SNR, right side, middle) at a specified number of frequency bands.

● Auditory brainstem response (ABR) is electrical brain wave activity that is produced by the auditory brainstem in response to sound introduced to the baby's ears. The responses are recorded by a computer and evaluated to determine whether the auditory system is responding as expected to the sound.

Like OAEs, ABR testing is painless and can be done in a matter of minutes while the infant sleeps.

● Place surface electrodes on the baby's scalp and measure the ABRs.

In normal hearing infants, responses can generally be obtained within approximately 10 to 20 dB HL of behavioral thresholds.

Thus, if a response is present at the typical screening level of 35 dB HL, the baby would pass the screening and would be considered to have normal hearing.

Figure 2.

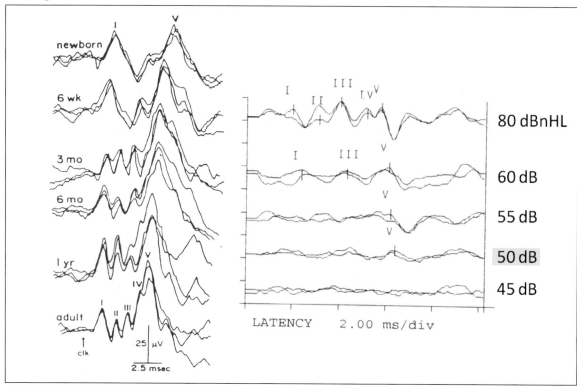

Source: Hall JW. *Handbook of Auditory Evoked Responses*. Boston, MA: Allyn & Bacon; 1992

Source: Ann Clock Eddins, PhD, CCC-A

The left panel of Figure 2 shows a series of ABRs as a function of age. Note the change in the number of peaks that can be identified as well as the decrease in latency of the peaks with age, resulting from neural maturation.[15]

The right panel of Figure 2 illustrates an ABR threshold series obtained from a child with sensorineural hearing loss using click stimuli. Threshold is estimated at 50 dBnHL, as indicated by the highlighted text.[16]

Screening for Hearing Loss in Toddlers and Young Children

Although studies have shown that only 50% of children with hearing loss are identified by the comprehensive use of risk assessment questionnaires, the National Institute on Deafness and Other Communication Disorders has published screening questions for children (>7 years) and adults, which are used in Bright Futures for risk assessment.

- Risk assessment questions (used for nonuniversal screening ages)

  ▶ Do you have a problem hearing over the telephone?

▶ Do you have trouble following the conversation when two or more people are talking at the same time?

▶ Do people complain that you turn the TV volume up too high?

▶ Do you have to strain to understand conversation?

▶ Do you have trouble hearing in a noisy background?

▶ Do you find yourself asking people to repeat themselves?

▶ Do many people you talk to seem to mumble (or not speak clearly)?

▶ Do you misunderstand what others are saying and respond inappropriately?

▶ Do you have trouble understanding the speech of women and children?

▶ Do people get annoyed because you misunderstand what they say?

Figure 3.

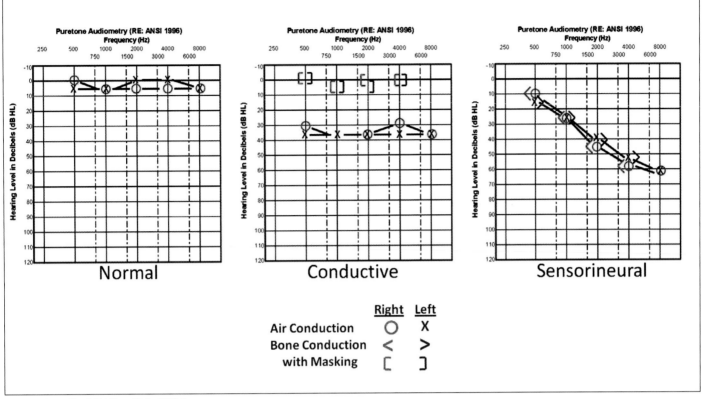

Source: Ann Clock Eddins, PhD, CCC-A

If there is a positive on the risk assessment questions, objective measures that can be used to screen for hearing loss and possible causes in toddlers and young children include OAE and ABR, as described previously, as well as behavioral pure tone audiometry and tympanometry.

- Behavioral pure tone audiometry is the standard for hearing evaluations. Different techniques are used depending on the age of the infant or child and his or her ability to follow directions or cooperate with the examination.

  ▶ Children 4 years or older often can be tested in a quiet room in a physician's office. Children younger than about 4 years generally can be tested more reliably by an audiologist in a sound-treated test booth rather than the physician's office.

  ▶ Each ear should be tested at 500, 1000, 2000, and 4000 Hz.

▶ Screening is typically done by presenting sounds at a fixed level of 20 or 25 dB HL across the frequency range, depending on the sound level in the room. If the child responds to sounds at that level, it is interpreted as a pass.

▶ If the child does not respond at any frequency, refer for a formal audiologic evaluation. If there is suspicion or concern about hearing loss, refer for further evaluation. Even a mild loss (25–40 dB HL) or a loss in one ear can result in delayed speech and language and academic development.

Figure 3 shows a series of audiograms illustrating normal hearing thresholds (left), conductive hearing loss (center), and sensorineural hearing loss (right).[17]

The degree of hearing loss is determined by measuring the dB HL required to just detect a tonal or noise signal 50% of the time. The scale in Figure 4 is used to define the degree of hearing loss.

Figure 4.

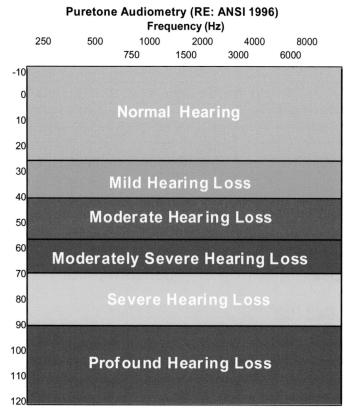

Puretone Audiometry (RE: ANSI 1996)

Source: Ann Clock Eddins, PhD, CCC-A

● Tympanometry is used to evaluate the function of the middle ear system. A small probe placed in the ear canal generates a low tone that changes with the air pressure in the ear canal. The resulting movement of the tympanic membrane and middle ear system is recorded. This test can be performed without any participation on the part of the child. The step-by-step protocol follows.

▶ Examine the ear otoscopically for evidence of external ear canal pathology, a perforated tympanic membrane, or pressure equalization or ventilation tube. Also examine for general size and shape.

▶ Instruct the patient about what you are about to do and ask her to sit quietly without responding to any sounds she might hear. Tell her to inform you if she feels any pain.

▶ Select a probe tip that is appropriate for the patient's ear canal and, gently pulling up and back on the pinna, insert the probe tip into the external ear canal with a slight twisting motion. Verify that the probe tip is well within the ear canal and filling the meatus.

▶ If you can't build up positive pressure, select another probe tip as appropriate and insert it into the ear canal.

▶ For automated tympanometers, simply press the start button to begin tympanometry.

▶ For manual equipment, increase pressure until you have reached +200 mmH20 (daPa).

▶ Plot the tympanogram or save it to a computer.

▶ Note important tympanogram findings, including ear canal volume, peak amplitude of the tympanogram, and pressure point of the peak.

Figure 5 provides examples of tympanograms used to evaluate the outer and middle ear systems. They are often classified based on their shape using the Jerger classification system. Type A shows a normal response. Type B shows a flat response, which is typically indicative

Figure 5.

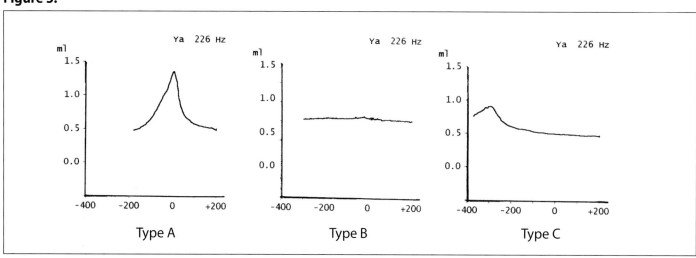

Source: Ann Clock Eddins, PhD, CCC-A

of OME. Type C shows a response with negative peak pressure, which is typically indicative of eustachian tube dysfunction.

What Should You Do With an Abnormal Result?

Conductive Hearing Loss

- Refer children with persistent conductive hearing loss to an otolaryngologist.

Sensorineural Hearing Loss

- Refer children with sensorineural hearing loss to an otolaryngologist to determine whether medical treatment is warranted and to an audiologist to determine appropriate rehabilitation. Audiologists will then work with other professionals (eg, early intervention caseworkers, speech-language pathologists, educators) to coordinate the necessary support services that the child may need.

- Children with sensorineural hearing loss can usually be helped with amplifying devices such as hearing aids and frequency modulated systems.

- For children with more severe to profound hearing loss, a cochlear implant may provide more benefit than hearing aids, as this device bypasses the inner ear and directly stimulates the auditory nerve.

CPT and CD-9-CM Codes	
92551	Screening test, pure tone, air only
92552	Pure tone audiometry (threshold); air only
92567	Tympanometry (impedance testing)
398.8	Other specified forms of hearing loss

The American Academy of Pediatrics publishes a complete line of coding publications, including an annual edition of *Coding for Pediatrics*. For more information on these excellent resources, visit the American Academy of Pediatrics Online Bookstore at **www.aap.org/bookstore/**.

Mixed Hearing Loss

- Refer children with a mixed loss to an otolaryngologist for medical evaluation and to an audiologist for rehabilitation.

Central Hearing Loss

- The recommended assessments for infants with auditory neuropathy spectrum disorder include a pediatric and developmental evaluation and history, referrals for an otologic evaluation (imaging of the cochlea and auditory nerve), medical genetics, an ophthalmologic assessment, a neurologic evaluation (assessment of peripheral and cranial nerve function), a communications assessment, and a referral to an audiologist to determine appropriate rehabilitation.

- Refer children with a central hearing loss to an otolaryngologist and an audiologist as well as a neurosurgeon and oncologist.

What Results Should You Document?

Document the results of a hearing screening in the infant or child's medical chart.

Resources

Articles

Bachmann KR, Arvedson JC. Early identification and intervention for children who are hearing impaired. *Pediatr Rev.* 1998;19:155–165

National Institute on Deafness and Other Communication Disorders. *Ten Ways to Recognize Hearing Loss.* Bethesda, MD: National Institutes of Health; 2006. NIH Publication No. 01-4913. http://www.nidcd.nih.gov/health/hearing/10ways.asp

Web Sites

American Speech-Language-Hearing Association: http://www.asha.org/

Boys Town National Research Hospital: http://babyhearing.org

Early Hearing Detection & Intervention (EHDI) Program Centers for Disease Control and Prevention: http://www.cdc.gov/ncbddd/ehdi

National Center for Hearing Assessment & Management

National Institute on Deafness and Other Communication Disorders:

National Institutes of Health: http://www.nidcd.nih.gov/

National Newborn Screening & Genetics Resource Center: http://genes-r-us.uthscsa.edu/resources/newborn/HearingScreening.htm

Utah State University: http://www.infanthearing.org/index.html

References

1. Bess FH, Dodd-Murphy J, Parker RA. Children with minimal sensorineural hearing loss: prevalence, educational performance, and functional status. *Ear Hear.* 1998;19(5):339–354

2. Yoshinaga-Itano C, Apuzzo ML. Identification of hearing loss after age 18 months is not early enough. *Am Ann Deaf.* 1998;143(5):380–387

3. Moeller MP. Early intervention and language development in children who are deaf and hard of hearing. *Pediatrics.* 2000;106(3):e43

4. Yoshinaga-Itano C. Early intervention after universal neonatal hearing screening: impact on outcomes. *Ment Retard Dev Disabil Res Rev.* 2003;9(4):252–266

5. Lieu JE. Speech-language and educational consequences of unilateral hearing loss in children. *Arch Otolaryngol Head Neck Surg.* 2004;130(5):524–530

6. Ruben RJ. A time frame of critical/sensitive periods of language development. *Acta Otolaryngol.* 1997;117(2):202–205

7. Ruben RJ, Wallace IF, Gravel J. Long-term communication deficiencies in children with otitis media during their first year of life. *Acta Otolaryngol.* 1997;117(2):206–207

8. Harrison M, Roush J, Wallace J. Trends in age of identification and intervention in infants with hearing loss. *Ear Hear.* 2003;24(1):89–95

9. Yoshinaga-Itano C, Apuzzo ML. The development of deaf and hard of hearing children identified early through the high-risk registry. *Am Ann Deaf.* 1998;143(5):416–424

10. Yoshinaga-Itano C, Sedey AL, Coulter DK, Mehl AL. Language of early- and later-identified children with hearing loss. *Pediatrics.* 1998;102(5):1161–1171

11. Hall JW III, Grose JH, Pillsbury HC. Long-term effects of chronic otitis media on binaural hearing in children. *Arch Otolaryngol Head Neck Surg.* 1995;121(8):847–852

12. Hall JW III, Grose JH, Dev MB, Drake AF, Pillsbury HC. The effect of otitis media with effusion on complex masking tasks in children. *Arch Otolaryngol Head Neck Surg.* 1998;124(8):892–896

13. Tos M. Epidemiology and natural history of secretory otitis. *Am J Otol.* 1984;5(6):459–462

14. Williamson I, Dunleavey GJ, Bain J, Robinson D. The natural history of otitis media with effusion—a three-year study of the incidence and prevalence of abnormal tympanograms in four South West Hampshire infant and first schools. *J Laryngol Otol.* 1994;108(11):930–934

15. Hall JW. *Handbook of Auditory Evoked Responses.* Boston, MA: Allyn & Bacon; 1992

16. Stapells DR. What are Auditory Evoked Potentials? The University of British Columbia School of Audiology and Speech Science Web Site. 2005. http://www.audiospeech.ubc.ca/haplab/aep.htm. Accessed April 12, 2006

17. Audiology Awareness Campaign. Sample Audiograms. Audiology Awareness Campaign Web Site. 1999. http://www.audiologyawareness.com/hearinfo_agramdem.asp. Accessed April 13, 2006

LYNN C. GARFUNKEL, MD
SUSANNE TANSKI, MD, MPH

IMMUNIZATIONS, NEWBORN SCREENING, AND CAPILLARY BLOOD TESTS

This chapter includes basic information on the most common procedures in pediatrics, including injections and capillary blood testing. The chapter covers immunizations (by subcutaneous or intramuscular injection), newborn metabolic screening (by heel stick), anemia and lead screening (by finger stick), and tuberculosis exposure screening (by intradermal injection). Immunizations may also be administered by oral or nasal routes. Also discussed are newborn screening results and follow-up.

Why Are Immunizations and Screening Blood Tests Important?

Immunizations. Childhood immunizations protect children from dangerous childhood diseases. Immunizations are required by states based on recommendations by the Centers for Disease Control and Prevention (CDC), the Advisory Committee on Immunization Practices, and the American Academy of Pediatrics (AAP). For review of the immunization schedule visit http://www.cdc.gov/vaccines/recs/schedules/child-schedule.htm.

Newborn screening. Newborn screening is a system involving the actual testing, follow-up, diagnostic testing, and disease management within the medical home. Screening is done to identify unrecognized disease or defect before clinical presentation, and in most states is performed in the hospital of birth prior to discharge. Newborn screenings are done using spots of blood on filter paper that undergo tandem mass spectrometry, isoelectric focusing, and high-performance liquid chromatography. There are specific circumstances that require additional testing within the pediatric office, including repeat testing at 1 to 2 weeks of age that is required by 9 states (AZ, CO, DE, NV, NM, OR, TX, UT, WY)

and recommended by several other states. Office-based systems should be developed to ensure that all infants have been screened, taking into account home births and, in some instances, parental refusal, and results managed appropriately. Prompt identification and follow-up of out-of-range results are required to prevent significant morbidity, mortality, and disability from disease. As the medical home practitioner and most often the first provider to obtain abnormal results from the newborn screening program, pediatricians must be familiar with the meaning of positive screens, subsequent diagnostic testing, and referrals. In addition, the pediatrician must recognize the possibility of false-negative results and subsequent disease later in life.

Guidelines for newborn screening are decided at the state level, based on federal suggestions distributed by the Secretary's Advisory Committee on Heritable Disorders in Newborns and Children. Pediatricians must be familiar with their individual state's policies and often adjoining states, as infant screening is dependent on the hospital of birth and not the state of residence. Most states screen for congenital hypothyroidism, congenital adrenal hyperplasia (CAH), phenylketonuria (PKU), galactosemia, maple syrup urine disease (MSUD), biotinidase deficiency, and hemoglobinopathies, as well as several other amino

SCREENING

137

acidopathies and many organic and fatty acid defects. The National Newborn Screening Status Report for state-by-state screening can be found at http://genes-r-us.uthscsa.edu/nbsdisorders.pdf. Newborn screening fact sheets published in *Pediatrics* (2006;118;934–963) can also be found online at www.pediatrics.org/cgi/content/full/118/3/1304) for many of the more common inborn errors.

Anemia screening. Anemia screening by finger stick blood samples is recommended by the AAP universally at the 12-month health supervision visit and as determined by risk at the 4-, 18-month and annual visits from age 2 to 21.

Lead screening. Lead screening is also performed by finger stick blood sample and is recommended at the 12- and 24-month health supervision visit either by risk assessment or screening as appropriate, based on the universal screening requirement for patients with Medicaid or locale in high-prevalence areas. Risk assessment (questions provided below) for lead screening is also recommended multiple times during infancy, middle childhood, and adolescence. Refer to the AAP "Recommendations for Preventive Pediatric Health Care" available at: brightfutures.aap.org/clinicalpractice.html.

Tuberculosis exposure screening. The tuberculin test is done if a child is determined to be high risk by risk assessment questions as outlined in Bright Futures.

How Should You Perform These Procedures?

Immunizations

All subcutaneous and intramuscular injections should be to the appropriate depth in order to maximize immune response and minimize discomfort and side effects. The recommended depths of injection and needle length are demonstrated in Figures 1 and 2.

Subcutaneous Injection

- Sites include upper outer arm or outer aspect of upper thigh.

- Clean the area to be injected with alcohol.

- Insert the needle into subcutaneous tissue at a 45-degree angle then inject vaccine.

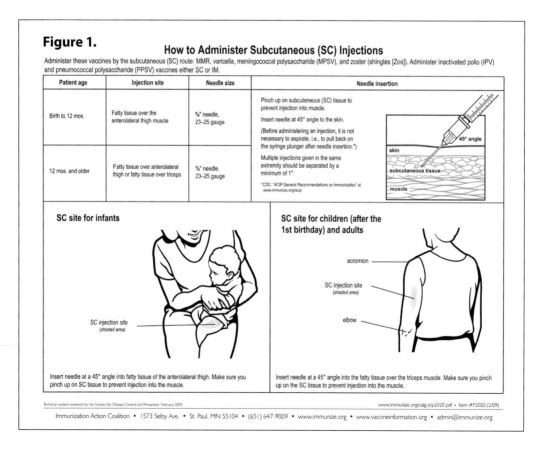

Figure 1.

How to Administer Subcutaneous (SC) Injections

Administer these vaccines by the subcutaneous (SC) route: MMR, varicella, meningococcal polysaccharide (MPSV), and zoster (shingles [Zos]). Administer inactivated polio (IPV) and pneumococcal polysaccharide (PPSV) vaccines either SC or IM.

Patient age	Injection site	Needle size	Needle insertion
Birth to 12 mos.	Fatty tissue over the anterolateral thigh muscle	⅝" needle, 23–25 gauge	Pinch up on subcutaneous (SC) tissue to prevent injection into muscle. Insert needle at 45° angle to the skin. (Before administering an injection, it is not necessary to aspirate, i.e., to pull back on the syringe plunger after needle insertion.*)
12 mos. and older	Fatty tissue over anterolateral thigh or fatty tissue over triceps	⅝" needle, 23–25 gauge	Multiple injections given in the same extremity should be separated by a minimum of 1". *CDC. "ACIP General Recommendations on Immunization" at www.immunize.org/acip

SC site for infants

Insert needle at a 45° angle into fatty tissue of the anterolateral thigh. Make sure you pinch up on SC tissue to prevent injection into the muscle.

SC site for children (after the 1st birthday) and adults

acromion

SC injection site *(shaded area)*

elbow

Insert needle at a 45° angle into the fatty tissue over the triceps muscle. Make sure you pinch up on the SC tissue to prevent injection into the muscle.

Technical content reviewed by the Centers for Disease Control and Prevention, February 2009.

www.immunize.org/catg.d/p2020.pdf • Item #P2020 (2/09)

Immunization Action Coalition • 1573 Selby Ave. • St. Paul, MN 55104 • (651) 647-9009 • www.immunize.org • www.vaccineinformation.org • admin@immunize.org

Figure 2. How to Administer Intramuscular (IM) Injections

Administer these vaccines by the intramuscular (IM) route: Diphtheria-tetanus (DT, Td) with pertussis (DTaP, Tdap); *Haemophilus influenzae* type b (Hib); hepatitis A (HepA); hepatitis B (HepB); human papillomavirus (HPV); inactivated influenza (TIV); meningococcal conjugate (MCV); and pneumococcal conjugate (PCV). Administer inactivated polio (IPV) and pneumococcal polysaccharide (PPSV) either IM or SC.

Patient age	Injection site	Needle size	Needle insertion
Newborn (0–28 days)	Anterolateral thigh muscle	⅝"* (22–25 gauge)	Use a needle long enough to reach deep into the muscle.
Infant (1–12 months)	Anterolateral thigh muscle	1" (22–25 gauge)	Insert needle at a 90° angle to the skin with a quick thrust.
Toddler (1–2 years)	Anterolateral thigh muscle	1–1¼" (22–25 gauge)	(Before administering an injection, it is not necessary to aspirate, i.e., to pull back on the syringe plunger after needle insertion.¶)
	Alternate site: Deltoid muscle of arm if muscle mass is adequate	⅝–1"* (22–25 gauge)	
Children (3–18 years)	Deltoid muscle	⅝–1"* (22–25 gauge)	Multiple injections given in the same extremity should be separated by a minimum of 1", if possible.
	Alternate site: Anterolateral thigh muscle	1–1¼" (22–25 gauge)	
Adults 19 years and older	Deltoid muscle of arm	1–1½"*† (22–25 gauge)	
	Alternate site: Anterolateral thigh muscle	1–1¼" (22–25 gauge)	

*A ⅝" needle may be used only if the skin is stretched tight, the subcutaneous tissue is not bunched, and injection is made at a 90° angle.
†A ⅝" needle is sufficient in adults weighing <130 lbs (<60 kg); a 1" needle is sufficient in adults weighing 130–152 lbs (60–70 kg); a 1–1½" needle is recommended in women weighing 152–200 lbs (70–90 kg) and men weighing 152–260 lbs (70–118 kg); a 1½" needle is recommended in women weighing >200 lbs (>90 kg) or men weighing >260 lbs (>118 kg).

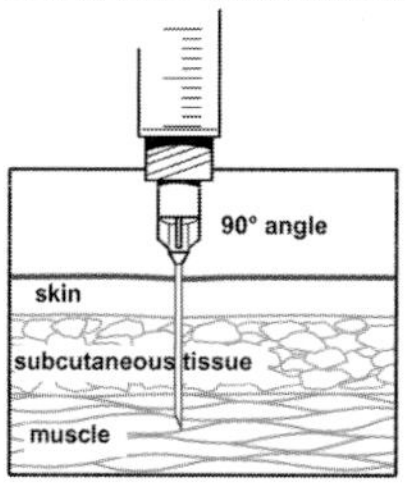

¶CDC. "ACIP General Recommendations on Immunization" at www.immunize.org/acip

90° angle
skin
subcutaneous tissue
muscle

IM site for infants and toddlers

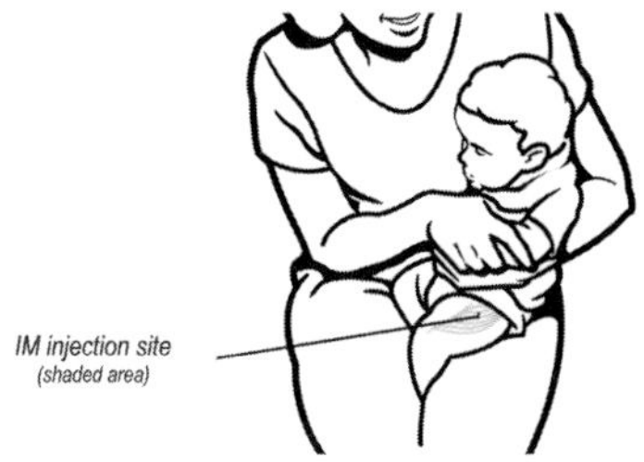

IM injection site (shaded area)

Insert needle at a 90° angle into the anterolateral thigh muscle.

IM site for children (after the 3rd birthday) and adults

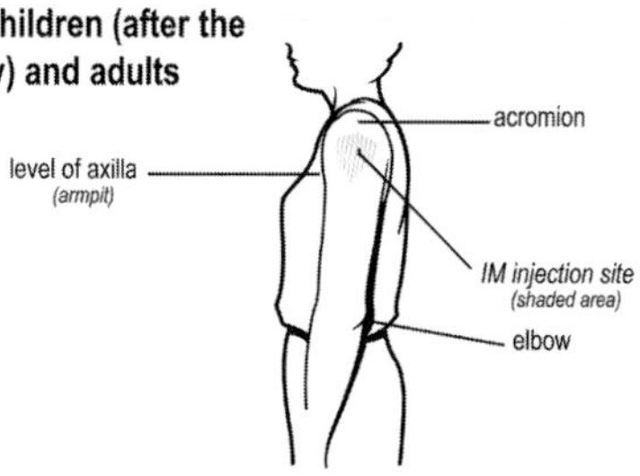

acromion
level of axilla (armpit)
IM injection site (shaded area)
elbow

Insert needle at a 90° angle into thickest portion of deltoid muscle — above the level of the axilla and below the acromion.

Technical content reviewed by the Centers for Disease Control and Prevention, February 2009.

www.immunize.org/catg.d/p2020.pdf • Item #P2020 (2/09)

Immunization Action Coalition • 1573 Selby Ave. • St. Paul, MN 55104 • (651) 647-9009 • www.immunize.org • www.vaccineinformation.org • admin@immunize.org

Intramuscular (IM) Injection

● Sites include the deltoid muscle of the upper arm for older children/adolescents or the vastus lateralis muscle in the anterolateral upper thigh for small children.

● Volumes for each IM injection are limited by age of child

  ▸ 0.5 mL for small infants

  ▸ 1 mL for larger infants

  ▸ 2 mL for school-aged children

  ▸ 3 mL for adolescents

● Clean the area to be injected with alcohol.

● Insert the needle to the appropriate depth, then inject vaccine.

As immunization recommendations are updated annually, current schedules may be obtained at the Web sites for the CDC (www.cdc.gov) or the AAP (www.aap.org).

Newborn Screening

Use a heel stick procedure for this test.

● Warm the heel with a warm compress for several minutes before sampling.

● Clean the area with alcohol.

● Using a sterile medical lancet, puncture the heel on the lateral aspect, avoiding the posterior area. Or, puncture the finger on the ventral lateral surface near the tip.

● Wipe away the first drop of blood with dry gauze, then collect blood on absorbent filter paper.

Anemia and Lead Screening

Anemia Risk

Infancy

● Prematurity

● Low birth weight

- Use of low-iron formula or infants not receiving iron-fortified formula

- Early introduction of cow's milk as a major source of nutrition. If infants are not yet consuming a sufficient alternate source of iron-rich foods, replacement of breast milk or formula may lead to insufficient iron intake.

Early and Middle Childhood (ages 18 month–5 years)

- At risk of iron deficiency because of special health needs

- Low-iron diet (eg, nonmeat diet)

- Environmental factors (eg, poverty, limited access to food)

Middle Childhood (6–10 years)

- Strict vegetarian diet and not receiving an iron supplement

Adolescence (11–21 years)

- Extensive menstrual or other blood loss

- Low iron intake

- Previously diagnosed with iron-deficiency anemia

Lead Risk

Lead Exposure Risk Assessment Questions

- For children ages 9 months to 6 years, ask screening questions for lead exposure[4]:

  ▷ Does your child live in or regularly visit a house or child care facility built before 1950?

  ▷ Does your child live in or regularly visit a house or child care facility built before 1978 that is being or has recently been renovated or remodeled (within the last 6 months)?

  ▷ Does your child have a sibling or playmate who has or did have lead poisoning?

- Perform finger stick/heel stick procedure.

  ▷ Warm the heel or finger with a warm compress for several minutes before sampling.

  ▷ Clean the area with alcohol.

  ▷ Using a sterile medical lancet, puncture the heel on the lateral aspect avoiding the posterior area. Or, puncture the finger on the ventral lateral surface near the tip.

  ▷ Wipe away the first drop of blood with a dry gauze, then collect blood with capillary tube/container. Avoid "milking" capillary stick site, as this increases tissue fluid in the sample and may falsely lower the result.

Tuberculosis Screening

- Every 6 months until age 2 years, then annually, ask the following screening questions for tuberculosis exposure[5]:

  ▷ Has a family member or contact had tuberculosis disease?

  ▷ Has a family member had a positive tuberculin skin test?

  ▷ Was your child born in a high-risk country (countries other than the United States, Canada, Australia, New Zealand, or Western European countries)?

  ▷ Has your child traveled to, and had contact with resident populations of, a high-risk country for more than 1 week?

- For those at high risk of disease, perform tuberculosis screening by intradermal injection of 0.5 mL of purified protein derivative (PPD).

  ▷ Clean volar surface of left or right forearm with alcohol. Let it dry.

  ▷ Wipe stopper of PPD vial with another alcohol pad. Let it dry.

  ▷ Draw 0.1 cc of PPD (5TU) into syringe, and with needle bevel up, inject full 0.1 cc into volar aspect of mid-forearm intradermally (just beneath the surface of the skin) so that a 5- to 10-mm wheal is created.

- Obtain results between 48 and 72 hours after injection.

  ▷ With arm flexed, feel for induration at the site of injection.

  ▷ To aid in measurement, using a ballpoint pen, mark the arm by moving the pen toward the induration, stopping at the point of induration/resistance.

- Draw lines from both directions (vertically and horizontally).

- Measure the induration with a millimeter ruler transversely to the long axis of the arm.

- Do not measure or record erythema without any induration (ie, erythema without any induration = 0 mm of induration).

What Should You Do With an Abnormal Result?

Newborn Metabolic and Hemoglobinopathy Screen

Manage abnormalities based on the specific abnormality. Newborn screening results are, in general, considered "in range," "out of range," or "invalid." States vary in screening guidelines and recommendations (see above). The AAP has endorsed the work of the American College of Medical Genetics (ACMG) and in 2006 published a technical report "Introduction to the Newborn Screening Fact Sheets" by Celia I. Kaye, MD, PhD, and the AAP Committee on Genetics (*Pediatrics,* 2006;118[3];1304–1312). The newborn screening information includes not only a description of the newborn test, but importantly the follow-up of abnormal screening results. Systematic follow-up is required to facilitate timely diagnostic testing and management, as well as the diagnostic tests and disease management (including coordination of care and genetic counseling). The following disorders are reviewed in the newborn screening fact sheets (which are available at www.pediatrics.org/cgi/content/full/118/3/e934): biotinidase deficiency, CAH, congenital hypothyroidism, cystic fibrosis, galactosemia, homocystinuria, MSUD, medium-chain acyl-coenzyme A dehydrogenase deficiency, PKU, sickle cell disease and other hemoglobinopathies, and tyrosinemia. While not a metabolic disease, information on congenital hearing loss is also available from the ACMG.

You must know what is screened for in your state. Many states have centrally located referral centers for medical care for specific abnormalities, which can also be accessed on the ACMG site.

- Pediatric endocrinology for abnormal CAH and thyroid screen

- Pediatric genetics for the range of inborn errors of metabolism, including PKU, MSUD, galactosidase, and other amino acid defects as well as biotinidase deficiency and fatty acid and organic acid abnormalities

- Pediatric pulmonology for cystic fibrosis

- Pediatric hematology for abnormal hemoglobin electrophoretic patterns

In many cases of abnormal screening, further confirmatory testing is necessary before a diagnosis is reached. The pediatrician may choose to do these tests or have them done by the referral center. The ACMG provides a free service for many of the common newborn screening tests. Included is a description of condition, a brief reference for differential diagnosis, actions to be taken, diagnostic evaluation, clinical considerations, reporting requirements, and links to additional resources, all easily accessed http://www.acmg.net/AM/Template.cfm?Section=NBS_ACT_Sheets_and_Algorithms_Table&Template=/CM/HTMLDisplay.cfm&ContentID=5072.

Lead or Anemia Screening

Abnormal lead results will need further workup and treatment, such as lead avoidance, possibly abatement, and potentially chelation.

For abnormal anemia results see Table 1, iron replenishment and supplementation may be the first and only step. However, it is important to determine whether abnormalities continue or whether other etiologies exist that warrant further investigation and treatment.

Tuberculosis Exposure Screening

Clinical factors will determine which size PPD (≥5 mm, ≥10 mm, or ≥15 mm) is positive (see AAP 2009 *Redbook,* page 681, Table 3.79 Definitions of Positive Tuberculin Skin Test Results in Infants, Children, and Adolescents). Those with positive PPDs need to have a chest x-ray. In most districts, public health authorities will need to be informed, and follow-up with pediatric pulmonology or infectious disease specialists may be warranted if chest x-ray is abnormal.

Changes in therapeutic recommendations may occur, thus the most recent AAP *Red Book* should be consulted or a referral made to a consulting tuberculosis specialist. The 2009 AAP *Red Book* recommends the following treatments:

Table 1. Fifth Percentile Cutoffs for Various Measures of Iron Deficiency in Childhood

Age, y	Hgb, g/dL	Hct, %	MCV, fL	ZnPP µg/dL	RDW, %	%TIBC saturation	Ferritin, µg/L
Newborn	<14.0	<42	NA	NA	NA	NA	<40
0.5–2.0	<11.0	<32.9	<77	>80	>14	<16	<15
2.0–4.9	<11.1	<33.0	<79	>70	>14	<16	<15
5.0–7.9	<11.5	<34.5	<80	>70	>14	<16	<15
8.0–11.9	<11.9	<35.4	<80	>70	>14	<16	<15
12.0–15.0 (male)	<12.5	<37.3	<82	>70	>14	<16	<15
12.0–15.0 (female)	<11.8	<35.7	<82	>70	>14	<16	<15
>15.0 (male)	<13.3	<39.7	<85	>70	>14	<16	<15
>15.0 (female)	<12.0	<35.7	<85	>70	>14	<16	<15

Abbreviations: Hct, hematocrit concentration; Hgb; hemoglobin concentration; MCV, mean corpuscular volume; NA, not applicable (no standards available); RDW, red blood cell distribution width; %TIBC, percent total iron-binding capacity; ZnPP, zinc protoporphyrin concentration.

Source: Reproduced from Kleinman, RE (2009) Pediatric Nutrition Handbook, 6th Edition, Elk Grove Village, IL

Latent tuberculosis (positive skin test, no disease)

- Isoniazid (INH)-susceptible: 9 months of INH, daily. If daily is not possible, direct observation of therapy (DOT) 2 times/week for 9 months.

- INH-resistant: 6 months rifampin, once daily. If daily is not possible, DOT 2 times/week for 6 months.

- INH-rifampin resistant: Consult tuberculosis specialist.

Pulmonary and extrapulmonary

- 2 months INH, rifampin and pyrazinamide daily, followed by 4 months INH and rifampin by direct observation of therapy for drug-susceptible *Mycobacterium tuberculosis*. Ideally, treatment is daily for first 2 weeks to 2 months, then 2 to 3 times per week by DOT.

- Extend duration to 9 months if initial chest x-ray shows cavitary lesions and sputum after 2 months of treatment is positive. If hilar adenopathy, only 6 months duration probably sufficient. Meds given 2 or 3 times/week under DOT in initial phase if nonadherence likely.

- 9 to 12 months of INH and rifampin for drug susceptible *Mycobacterium bovis*.

Meningitis

- 2 months INH, rifampin, pyrazinamide, and an aminoglycoside or ethionamide daily; followed by 7 to 10 months of isoniazid and rifampin daily or 2times/week (9–12 months total) for drug-susceptible M.TB

- At least 12 months without pyrazinamide for drug-susceptible *M Bovis*.

- Give a fourth drug—aminoglycoside—with initial treatment until susceptibility is known.

What Results Should We Document?

Immunizations

Document the immunization procedure (injection type, site, manufacturer, lot number and expiration of vaccine, provision of Vaccine Information Statement). Record all immunizations in the medical record. In some states, immunizations must also be recorded in a state registry.

Newborn Metabolic Screen

Make results of the newborn metabolic screen available in the patient chart. Note documentation of discussion of normal and abnormal results. Document parental refusal.

Include referral to appropriate center (or documentation of plan), or repeat or further lab testing, for those infants who have abnormal, questionable, or invalid results.

Lead and Anemia Screening

Document results of lead levels and hematocrit in the patient chart. In some practices this is noted in the specific visit record. Many medical records have an easily accessible section, chart, or graph for recording all screening test results and immunizations.

Tuberculosis Exposure Screen

Document the PPD procedure (injection type, site, lot number, and expiration of PPD). Record result of testing (including measurement of area of induration) in the medical record.

ICD-9-CM and *CPT* Codes

Immunizations

There are separate billing codes for the vaccine product, administration of the vaccine, and for patient evaluation and management services. Advice on *CPT* coding should be obtained as needed, as codes and rules for coding do change regularly.

The *ICD-9-CM* codes for vaccine administration: "Inoculations and vaccinations: Categories V03–V06 are for encounters for inoculations and vaccinations. They indicate that a patient is being seen to receive a prophylactic inoculation against a disease. The injection itself must be represented by the appropriate procedure code. A code from V03–V06 may be used as a secondary code if the inoculation is given as a routine part of preventive health care, such as a well-baby visit."[3]

The *CPT* codes are classified by vaccination and available at http://www.aap.org/immunization/pediatricians/pdf/VaccineCodingTable.pdf.

Codes 99381–99385 are evaluation and management (E/M) codes for an office or outpatient visit for the initial comprehensive preventive E/M of a patient. Codes 99391–99395 are E/M codes for established patients for periodic comprehensive preventive visit.

Code 90471 is for immunization administration (includes percutaneous, intradermal, subcutaneous, IM and jet injections), one vaccine (single or combination vaccine/toxoid). Code 90473 is for immunization by intranasal or oral route (single vaccine).

Code 90472 is for each additional vaccine (single or combination vaccine). (List separately in addition to the code for primary procedure.) Code 90474 is for each additional intranasal or oral vaccine.

When counseling for immunization administration that does not include a visit, well-child care, or an illness, but the physician provides face-to-face counseling to the family, the following codes are used for children younger than 8: 90465—percutaneous, intradermal, subcutaneous, IM, and jet injections, one vaccine (single or combination vaccine/toxoid)); 90466—each additional vaccine; 90467—initial intranasal or oral vaccine; 90468 for each additional intranasal or oral immunization.

Newborn Screening

The *CPT* code for newborn screen retesting is 84030, and the diagnosis code is 270.10.

Screening Procedures

- Heel stick blood draw CPT 36416—Collection of capillary blood specimen (finger, ear, heel stick)

- Finger stick blood draw *CPT* 36416—Collection of capillary blood specimen (finger, ear, heel stick)

- PPD—intradermal *CPT* 86580 (skin test; tuberculosis, intradermal)

Resources

Newborn screen disease descriptions for parents and physicians (also has multiple language translations).

Save Babies Through Screening Foundation Inc.: http://www.savebabies.org/disease_descriptions.html

Articles

1. Groswasser J, Kahn A, Bouche B, Hanquinet S, Perlmuter N, Hessel L. Experience and reason: needle length and injection technique for efficient intramuscular vaccine delivery in infants and children evaluated through an ultrasonographic determination of subcutaneous and muscle layer thickness. *Pediatrics.* 1997;100(3):400–403

2. Cook IF, Murtagh J. The consultation research: optimal technique for intramuscular injection of infants and toddlers: a randomised trial. *Med J Aust.* 2005;183(2):60–63

3. American Medical Association. *CPT: Current Procedural Terminology.* Chicago, IL: American Medical Association; 2009

4. American Academy of Pediatrics Committee on Environmental Health. Screening for elevated blood lead levels. *Pediatrics.* 1998;101:1072–1078

5. American Academy of Pediatrics. Tuberculosis. In: Pickering LK, Baker CJ, Kimberlin DW, Long SS, eds. *Red Book: 2009 Report of the Committee on Infectious Diseases.* 28th ed. Elk Grove Village, IL: American Academy of Pediatrics; 2009:680–681

6. National Newborn Screening Status Report. National Newborn Screening and Genetics Resource Center Web Site. 2009. http://genes-r-us.uthscsa.edu/nbsdisorders.pdf

7. Kaye CI; American Academy of Pediatrics Committee on Genetics. Introduction to the newborn screening fact sheets. *Pediatrics.* 2006;118(3):1304–1312. http://www.pediatrics.org/cgi/content/full/118/3/e934

8. Newborn Screening Authoring Committee. Newborn screening expands: recommendations for pediatricians and medical homes: implications for the system. *Pediatrics.* 2008;121;192–217. http://www.pediatrics.org/cgi/doi/10.1542/peds.2007-3021

Web Sites

American College of Medical Genetics Newborn screening ACT and confirmatory algorithms: http://www.acmg.net/AM/Template.cfm?Section=NBS_ACT_Sheets_and_Algorithms_Table&Template=/CM/HTMLDisplay.cfm&ContentID=5072

Centers for Disease Control and Prevention: http://www.cdc.gov/vaccines/recs/schedules/child-schedule.htm Vaccine schedules.

Medline Plus: http://www.nlm.nih.gov/medlineplus/newbornscreening.html
Newborn screen disease descriptions for parents and physicians.

National Newborn Screening & Genetics Resource Center: http://genes-r-us.uthscsa.edu
Newborn screening recommendations by state.

Newborn Screening Authoring Committee: www.pediatrics.org/cgi/doi/10.1542/peds.2007-3021
Newborn screening clinical report.

Administering Vaccines: Dose, Route, Site, and Needle Size

Vaccines	Dose	Route
Diphtheria, Tetanus, Pertussis (DTaP, DT, Tdap, Td)	0.5 mL	IM
Haemophilus influenzae type b (Hib)	0.5 mL	IM
Hepatitis A (HepA)	≤18 yrs: 0.5 mL ≥19 yrs: 1.0 mL	IM
Hepatitis B (HepB) *Persons 11–15 yrs may be given Recombivax HB® (Merck) 1.0 mL adult formulation on a 2-dose schedule.	≤19 yrs: 0.5 mL* ≥20 yrs: 1.0 mL	IM
Human papillomavirus (HPV)	0.5 mL	IM
Influenza, live attenuated (LAIV)	0.5 mL	Intranasal spray
Influenza, trivalent inactivated (TIV)	6–35 mos: 0.25 mL ≥3 yrs: 0.5 mL	IM
Measles, mumps, rubella (MMR)	0.5 mL	SC
Meningococcal – conjugate (MCV)	0.5 mL	IM
Meningococcal – polysaccharide (MPSV)	0.5 mL	SC
Pneumococcal conjugate (PCV)	0.5 mL	IM
Pneumococcal polysaccharide (PPSV)	0.5 mL	IM or SC
Polio, inactivated (IPV)	0.5 mL	IM or SC
Rotavirus (RV)	2.0 mL	Oral
Varicella (Var)	0.5 mL	SC
Zoster (Zos)	0.65 mL	SC

Combination Vaccines

DTaP+HepB+IPV (Pediarix®) DTaP+Hib+IPV (Pentacel®) DTaP+Hib (Trihibit®) DTaP+IPV (Kinrix®) Hib+HepB (Comvax®)	0.5 mL	IM
MMR+Var (ProQuad®)	≤12 yrs: 0.5 mL	SC
HepA+HepB (Twinrix®)	≥18 yrs: 1.0 mL	IM

Injection Site and Needle Size

Subcutaneous (SC) injection Use a 23–25 gauge needle. Choose the injection site that is appropriate to the person's age and body mass.

Age	Needle Length	Injection Site
Infants (1–12 mos)	5/8"	Fatty tissue over anterolateral thigh muscle muscle
Children 12 mos or older, adolescents, & adults	5/8"	Fatty tissue over anterolateral thigh muscle or fatty tissue over triceps

Intramuscular (IM) injection Use a 22–25 gauge needle. Choose the injection site and needle length appropriate to the person's age and body mass.

Age	Needle Length	Injection Site
Newborn (1st 28 days)	5/8"	Anterolateral thigh muscle
Infants (1–12 mos)	1"	Anterolateral thigh muscle
Toddlers (1–2 yrs)	1"–1¼" 5/8–1"	Anterolateral thigh muscle or deltoid muscle of arm
Children & teens (3–18 years)	5/8–1"* 1"–1¼"	Deltoid muscle of arm or Anterolateral thigh muscle
Adults 19 yrs or older		
Male or Female less than 130 lbs	5/8–1"*	Deltoid muscle of arm
Female 130–200 lbs Male 130–260 lbs	1–1½"	Deltoid muscle of arm
Female 200+ lbs Male 260+ lbs	1½"	Deltoid muscle of arm

*A 5/8" needle may be used only if the skin is stretched tight, subcutaneous tissue is not bunched, and injection is made at a 90-degree angle.

Please note: Always refer to the package insert included with each biologic for complete vaccine administration information. CDC's Advisory Committee on Immunization Practices (ACIP) recommendations for the particular vaccine should be reviewed as well.

Technical content reviewed by the Centers for Disease Control and Prevention, Nov. 2006. www.immunize.org/catg.d/p3085.pdf • Item #P3085 (11/15/06)

Source: Immunization Action Coalition • 1573 Selby Ave. • St. Paul, MN 55104 • (651) 647-9009 • www.immunize.org • www.vaccineinformation.org

SCREENING

145

SUSAN M. YUSSMAN, MD, MPH

SEXUALLY TRANSMITTED INFECTIONS

Why Is It Important to Screen for Sexually Transmitted Infections?

Sexually transmitted infections (STIs) are common. Every year, 19 million STIs occur. Almost half occur in youth aged 15 to 24. One in 4 sexually active adolescents will be infected with an STI by age 21. The prevalence of chlamydia in women aged 14 to 19 years is nearly 5%, the highest proportion of any age group.

Adolescents are at high risk. There are now more than 20 STIs. Adolescents are at high risk of STIs due to cervical ectopy (columnar epithelium present on the cervix), immature immune system, multiple partners, inconsistent condom use, and barriers to health care.

Sexually transmitted infections have high costs. Sexually transmitted infections in youth pose an economic burden of $15.5 billion a year.

Sexually transmitted infections often have no symptoms and therefore go undiagnosed, leading to disease. In women, a spectrum of diseases exist, including vulvovaginitis, vaginitis, cervicitis, endometritis, salpingitis, tubo-ovarian abscess, and peritonitis. In men, the spectrum of disease includes urethritis, epididymitis, and prostatitis. If left untreated, STIs can cause severe health consequences, including pelvic inflammatory disease, epididymitis, ectopic pregnancy, infertility, cervical cancer, and death.

Sexually transmitted infection screening is recommended. The Centers for Disease Control and Prevention recommends annual chlamydia screening for all sexually active women younger than 25.

Bright Futures recommends screening all sexually active youth for gonorrhea and chlamydia annually. For high-risk teens, also screen for syphilis and HIV at least once a year. For high-risk teens, STI testing, especially for chlamydia, may be done as often as every 3 to 6 months. High-risk teens include, but are not limited to, STI clinic patients, youth in detention centers, men who have sex with men, and injection drug users. Other STIs should be screened for only if a patient is symptomatic. For instance, if a patient has a genital ulcer, then add a herpes culture to the evaluation. If a patient has cervicitis, then conduct additional testing for trichomoniasis.

How Should You Perform STI Screening?

Take a Detailed Sexual History

Ask about

- Age at first intercourse
- Number of sex partners
- Sex with males, females, or both
- Types of sex (oral, vaginal, anal)
- Sexual orientation
- Use of barrier and hormonal contraception
- Prior STI testing and results
- History of sexual abuse

Perform Screening

In all states and the District of Columbia, adolescents are able to consent to diagnosis and treatment of STIs. Most states also allow adolescents to consent for confidential HIV counseling and testing.

SCREENING

Chlamydia and Gonorrhea

- Nucleic acid amplification tests

  ▸ Amplify and detect organism-specific genomic or plasmid DNA or rRNA

  ▸ Polymerase chain reaction

  ▸ Transcription-mediated amplification

  ▸ Strand displacement amplification

Trichomoniasis

- Nucleic acid amplification tests testing-urine sample or vaginal/endocervical swab sample

- Wet prep-vaginal swab sample

- Motile trichomonads seen on saline wet mount

- Vaginal pH >4.5 and positive amine whiff test help confirm the diagnosis, but are also seen with bacterial vaginosis

- Other point-of-care testing-vaginal swab sample

- Antigen detection test

- Nucleic acid probe-hybridization test

- Culture

Genital Warts (Human Papillomavirus [HPV])

- Visual inspection with bright light.

- Can be confirmed by biopsy

- Use of type-specific HPV DNA tests for routine diagnosis and management of genital warts is not recommended.

Herpes

- Viral culture of fluid from an unroofed pustule is best because sensitivity of culture declines rapidly as lesions begin to heal.

- Herpes simplex virus-2 serologic tests are not indicated for screening in the general population, but can be used to confirm a clinical diagnosis or to diagnose persons with unrecognized infection.

Syphilis

- Darkfield examination and direct fluorescent antibody tests of lesion exudates are definitive.

- Serologic tests

  ▸ Nontreponemal tests

    - Venereal Disease Research Laboratory

    - Rapid plasma reagin

    - Most reactive tests become nonreactive after treatment

  ▸ Treponemal tests

    - Fluorescent treponemal antibody absorbed

    - *Treponema* pallidum particle agglutination

    - Most reactive tests always remain positive

HIV

- Serologic antibody testing with enzyme immunoassay

- Rapid oral or blood test which gives a result within 30 minutes is also acceptable for screening.

- All reactive screening tests must be confirmed by Western blot or immunofluorescence assay

- The HIV antibody is detectable in 95% of patients within 3 months after infection

What Should We Do With an Abnormal Result?

All sexual partners from the past 60 days of patients positive for chlamydia, gonorrhea, and trichomoniasis should be tested and treated, regardless of their test results. Sexual partners from the past 90 days of patients positive for primary syphilis should be tested and treated even if seronegative. Partners of those positive for HIV should be tested immediately, in one month, in 3 months, and in 6 months.

Treatments

Chlamydia cervicitis or urethritis

- Azithromycin 1 g orally in a single dose, OR

- Doxycycline 100 mg orally twice daily for 7 days

Gonorrhea cervicitis or urethritis

- Ceftriaxone 125 mg IM in a single dose, OR

- Cefixime 400 mg orally in a single dose

- Fluoroquinolones are no longer recommended due to resistance.

Pelvic Inflammatory Disease (cervical motion tenderness or adnexal tenderness)

- Ceftriaxone 250 mg IM in a single dose PLUS doxycycline 100 mg orally twice a day for 14 days WITH OR WITHOUT metronidazole 500 mg orally twice a day for 14 days OR

- Cefoxitin 2 g IM in a single dose and probenecid, 1 g orally administered concurrently in a single dose PLUS doxycycline 100 mg orally twice a day for 14 days WITH OR WITHOUT metronidazole 500 mg orally twice a day for 14 days

Trichomoniasis

- Metronidazole 2 g orally in a single dose OR

- Tinidazole 2 g orally single dose (non-pregnant patients only)

- Metronidazole 500 mg twice a day for 7 days OR

External Genital Warts

- Patient-Applied Treatments

  Choose **one** of the following treatment options:

  ▷ Podofilox 0.5% solution or gel to visible warts twice a day for 3 days, followed by 4 days of no therapy up to 4 cycles

  ▷ Imiquimod 5% cream once daily at bedtime, 3 times a week for up to 16 weeks (wash off 6–10 hours after application)

- Provider-Applied Treatments

  Choose **one** of the following treatment options:

  ▷ Cryotherapy with liquid nitrogen or cryoprobe every 1 to 2 weeks

  ▷ Podophyllin resin 10% to 25% in compound tincture of benzoin to each wart and air-dry, up to weekly if needed

▷ Trichloroacetic acid or bichlproacetic acid 80% to 90% to warts and air dry up to weekly

Genital Herpes

- First Clinical Episode

  Choose **one** of the following treatment options:

  ▷ Acyclovir 400 mg orally 3 times a day for 7 to 10 days

  ▷ Acyclovir 200 mg orally 5 times a day for 7 to 10 days

  ▷ Famciclovir 250 mg orally 3 times a day for 7 to 10 days

  ▷ Valacyclovir 1 g orally twice a day for 7 to 10 days

- Recurrent Episodes

  Choose **one** of the following treatment options:

  ▷ Acyclovir 400mg orally three times a day for 5 days

  ▷ Acyclovir 800mg orally twice a day for 5 days

  ▷ Acyclovir 800mg orally three times a day for 2 days

  ▷ Famciclovir 125mg orally twice daily for 5 days

  ▷ Famciclovir 10000mg orally twice daily for 1 day

  ▷ Valacyclovir 500mg orally twice a day for 3 days

  ▷ Valacyclovir 1000mg orally once a day for 5 days

- Daily Suppressive Therapy for Recurrent Herpes

  Choose **one** of the following treatment options:

  ▷ Acyclovir 400 mg orally twice a day

  ▷ Famciclovir 250 mg orally twice a day

  ▷ Valacyclovir 500 mg or 1 g orally once daily

Syphilis

- Primary and Secondary Syphilis

  ▷ Benzathine penicillin G 50,000 units/kg IM, up to the adult dose of 2.4 million units in a single dose

- Early latent syphilis (seroactivity conversion within prior year without other evidence of disease)

  ▷ Benzathine penicillin G 50,000 units/kg IM, up to the adult dose of 2.4 million units, administered as 3 doses at 1-week intervals (total 150,000units/kg up to the adult total dose of 7.2 million units)

- Late latent syphilis (seroactivity conversion more than 1 year prior or of unknown duration without other evidence of disease)

  ▶ Benzathine penicillin G 7.2 million units IM total, administered as 3 doses of 2.4 million units IM each at 1-week intervals

- Tertiary syphilis (gumma and cardiovascular syphilis)

  ▶ Benzathine penicillin G 7.2 million units IM total, administered as 3 doses of 2.4 million units IM each at 1-week intervals

What Results Should You Document?

As of 2010, all states mandate reporting of gonorrhea, chlamydia, syphilis, and HIV to local health departments.

Check with your local health department to determine if other STIs are reportable.

Resources

Books

Emans SJ, Laufer MR, Goldstein DP, eds. *Pediatric and Adolescent Gynecology*. 4th ed. Philadelphia, PA: Lippincott Williams & Wilkins; 1998

Fortenberry JD. Sexually transmitted infections: screening and diagnosis guidelines for primary care pediatricians. *Pediatr Ann*. 2005;34:803–810

Articles

Burstein GR, Murray PJ. Diagnosis and management of sexually transmitted disease pathogens among adolescents. *Pediatr Rev*. 2003;24:75–82

Burstein GR, Murray PJ. Diagnosis and management of sexually transmitted diseases among adolescents. *Pediatr Rev*. 2003;24:119–127

Centers for Disease Control and Prevention, Workowski KA, Berman SM. Sexually transmitted diseases treatment guidelines, 2006. *MMWR Recomm Rep*. 2006;55(RR-11):1–94

ICD-9-CM Codes	
131.00	Urogenital trichomoniasis unspecified site
131.01	Trichomoniasis vulvovaginitis
131.02	Trichomoniasis urethritis
131.03	Trichomoniasis prostatitis
098.0	Gonococcal urethritis
098.15	Gonococcal cervicitis
616.0	Cervictis
616.11	Vaginitis and vulvovaginitis
099.41	*Chlamydia trachomatis* urethritis
614.0	Pelvic inflammatory disease
054.10	Genital herpes
078.11	Genital warts
132.2	Pediculus pubis (pubic lice)
091.0	Genital syphilis
099.9	Venereal disease, unspecified
042	Human immunodeficiency virus disease
054.11	Herpetic vulvovaginitis
054.12	Herpetic ulceration of vulva
054.13	Herpetic ulceration of penis
054.2	Herpetic ginivostomatitis
099.40	Other non-gonococcal urethritis unspecified
099.50	Chlamydia unspecified site
099.51	Chlamydia pharyngitis
099.52	Chlamydia anus and rectum
091.0	Primary genital syphilis
091.1	Primary anal syphilis
091.2	Other primary syphilis
091.3	Secondary syphilis of skin or mucous membranes
091.4	Adenopathy due to secondary syphilis
614.9	Pelvic inflammatory disease not otherwise specified

The American Academy of Pediatrics publishes a complete line of coding publications, including an annual edition of *Coding for Pediatrics*. For more information on these excellent resources, visit the American Academy of Pediatrics Online Bookstore at **www.aap.org/bookstore/**.

Centers for Disease Control and Prevention, Division of STD Prevention, National Center for HIV/AIDS, Viral Hepatitis, STD and TB Prevention. Updated recommended treatment regimens for gonococcal infections and associated conditions—United States, April 2007. Centers for Disease Control and Prevention Web Site. 2007. http://www.cdc.gov/STD/treatment. Accessed August 21, 2007

Centers for Disease Control and Prevention. New data show heavy impact of Chlamydia on US men and women, particularly young people. Centers for Disease Control and Prevention Web Site. 2005. http://www.cdc.gov/media/pressrel/r050712.htm. Accessed June 4, 2010

Johnson RE, Newhall WJ, Papp JR. Screening tests to detect Chlamydia trachomatis and Neisseria gonorrhoeae infections—2002. MMWR Recomm Rep. 2002;51(RR15):1–27

Centers for Disease Control and Prevention, Division of STD Prevention, National Center for HIV/AIDS, Viral Hepatitis, STD and TB Prevention. Trends in reportable sexually transmitted diseases in the United States, 2003—national data on chlamydia, gonorrhea and syphilis. Centers for Disease Control and Prevention Web Site. 2004. http://www.cdc.gov/STD/stats03/trends2003.htm

Centers for Disease Control and Prevention, Division of STD Prevention, National Center for HIV/AIDS, Viral Hepatitis, STD and TB Prevention. Updated recommended treatment regimens for gonococcal infections and associated conditions—United States, April 2007. Centers for Disease Control and Prevention Web Site. 2007. http://www.cdc.gov/STD/treatment. Accessed August 21, 2007

Chesson HW, Blandford JM, Gift TL, Tao G, Irwin KL. The estimated direct medical cost of sexually transmitted diseases among American youth, 2000. Perspect Sex Reprod Health. 2004;36(1):11–19

Neinstein LS, ed. Adolescent Health Care: A Practical Guide. 4th ed. Philadelphia, PA: Lippincott Williams & Wilkins; 2002

Knight JR, Sherritt L, Shrier LA, Harris SK, Chang H. Validity of the CRAFFT Substance Abuse Screening Test among adolescent clinic patients. Arch Pediatr Adolesc Med. 2002;156:607–614

Weinstock H, Berman S, Cates W Jr. Sexually transmitted diseases among American youth: incidence and prevalence estimates, 2000. Perspect Sex Reprod Health. 2004;36:6–10

Web Sites for Health Professionals

CDC STI Treatment Guidelines: www.cdc.gov/std/treatment

Center for Young Women's Health at Boston Children's Hospital: www.youngwomenshealth.org

Web Sites for Adolescents and Parents

American Social Health Association: www.ashastd.org

Center for Young Women's Health at Boston Children's Hospital: www.youngwomenshealth.org

Nemours Foundation: www.kidshealth.org

Planned Parenthood: www.plannedparenthood.org

US Department of Health and Human Services: www.4women.gov

Reference

1. Guttmacher Institute. "State Policies in Brief: An overview of minors' Consent Law as of June 1, 2010. Available at: http://www.guttmacher.org/statecenter/spibs/sprb-omel.pdf

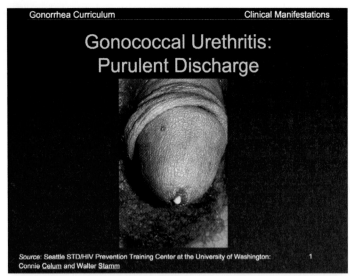

Gonorrhea Curriculum — Clinical Manifestations

Gonococcal Urethritis: Purulent Discharge

Source: Seattle STD/HIV Prevention Training Center at the University of Washington: Connie Celum and Walter Stamm

1

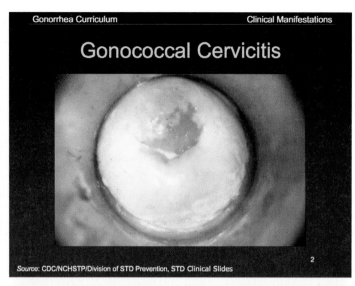

Gonorrhea Curriculum — Clinical Manifestations

Gonococcal Cervicitis

Source: CDC/NCHSTP/Division of STD Prevention, STD Clinical Slides

2

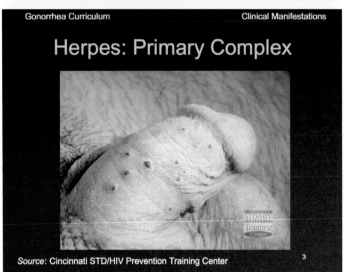

Gonorrhea Curriculum — Clinical Manifestations

Herpes: Primary Complex

Source: Cincinnati STD/HIV Prevention Training Center

3

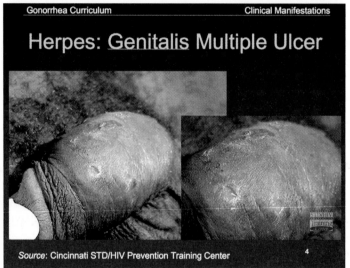

Gonorrhea Curriculum — Clinical Manifestations

Herpes: Genitalis Multiple Ulcer

Source: Cincinnati STD/HIV Prevention Training Center

4

Penile Warts

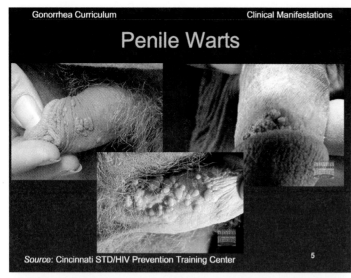

5

Perianal Warts

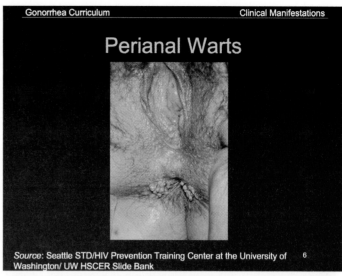

6

Primary Syphilis- Penile Chancre

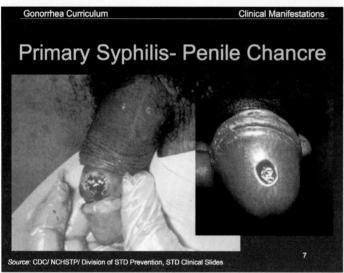

7

Secondary Syphilis: Palmar/Plantar Rash

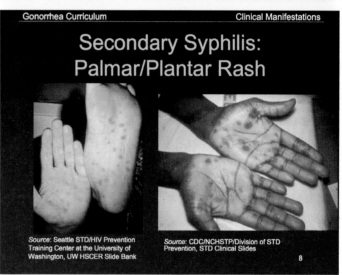

8

SCREENING

ALEX KEMPER, MD, MPH, MS
MONTE A. DELMONTE, MD

VISION

The goals of vision screening vary by the age of the child. For infants, the goals are to detect retinoblastoma, congenital glaucoma, and conditions that could lead to amblyopia if not detected early, such as congenital cataracts, ptosis, or significant strabismus. For preschool-aged children, the goals are to detect amblyopia and conditions that could lead to amblyopia (eg, strabismus and unequal refractive error between each eye and refractive error). For school-aged children, the goal is to detect refractive error.

Why Is It Important to Screen for Vision Problems?

Vision problems are common. Among preschool-aged children, 5% to 10% have vision problems, including 2% to 5% with strabismus or amblyopia. Among school-aged children and adolescent children, more than 10% have refractive errors, such as myopia or hyperopia.

Rare conditions present in infancy and early childhood. These conditions, which include congenital cataracts, congenital glaucoma, congenital ptosis, and retinoblastoma, can lead to blindness. Retinoblastoma can be fatal, and cataracts may be associated with other systemic disorders.

Early treatment leads to improved outcomes. The difficulty of treatment for amblyopia increases and the likelihood of cure decreases with increasing age of the child. Undetected congenital cataracts, glaucoma, or ptosis can lead to blindness in early infancy. Untreated refractive errors may affect learning.

Some children are at high risk of vision problems. Risk factors for vision problems include prematurity and family history of congenital cataracts or retinoblastoma. Special attention should be paid to children with special health care needs who may be difficult to screen, such as children with cerebral palsy or down syndrome.

When Should You Perform Vision Screening?

Assessing risk for ocular problems and vision impairment should begin in the newborn nursery and occur at all health supervision visits. Bright Futures recommends that all children have formal vision screening as part of their health supervision visit annually from 3 through 6 years of age, at 8 years of age, at 10 years of age, at 12 years of age, at 15 years of age, and at 18 years of age. Vision screening should be conducted at other health supervision visits based on risk assessment or any concern on the part of families or the child.

The American Academy of Pediatrics (AAP) recommends age-appropriate screening tests, which vary based on the goals across the age spectrum. Little is known about the accuracy of vision screening tests in the primary care practice setting, however.

Some children with vision problems appear to be uncooperative on testing. Follow-up testing in 1 to 6 months or referral is recommended if testing is equivocal or if the child is not cooperative.

SCREENING

How Should You Perform Vision Screening?

New vision screening technology (eg, photoscreening, autorefraction) has been developed and is increasingly used in pediatric practice. Reccomendations for the use of such technology will be made as evidence regarding their comparative effectiveness becomes available.

Birth to 3 Years

Assess for parent concern and ask for parent observations. Risk assessment must be adapted to the developmental status of the child. Examples of questions include:

- Does your child seem to see well?

- Does your child hold objects close to his or her face when trying to focus?

- Do your child's eyes appear unusual or do they seem to cross or drift or seem lazy?

- Do your child's eyelids droop or does one eyelid tend to close?

- Have your child's eyes ever been injured?

Take a family history. Explore relevant family histories about eye disorders, such as amblyopia, strabismus, congenital cataracts, retinoblastoma, or preschool or early childhood use of glasses in parents or siblings.

Conduct a physical examination. Assess ability to fix and follow.

- Inspect the eyes and lids.

- Evaluate ocular motility and alignment with the corneal light reflex test (Hirschberg test) and the cover/uncover and cross-cover tests. These tests can help identify strabisumus. Careful examination can also exclude psuedostrabismus. However, if there is doubt, refer to an eye care specialist.

- Examine the reaction of the pupils.

- Assess the red reflex for cataracts or leukocoria.

3 Years and Older

Assess for parent or child concern and ask for parent observations. Ask questions, such as

- Do you (or does your child) have trouble seeing the blackboard in the classroom?

- Do you (or does your child) hold toys or books close to the eyes?

- Do you (or does your child) have trouble recognizing faces at a distance?

- Do you (or does your child) tend to squint?

- Have you (or has your child) failed a school vision screening test?

Perform vision screening tests. This should include tests of distance visual acuity and tests of ocular alignment and stereovision.

- Distance visual acuity measurement for preschool-aged children (3–5 years)

  - Recommended charts include the HOTV chart and the Lea chart (heart, house, circle, square). Some children may be able to use the Snellen Chart.

  - All charts should be tested at 10 feet. If possible, consider testing within a quiet room and not in a heavily trafficked hallway.

- Test each eye individually. Make sure that the other eye is completely occluded.

  - Refer if less than 20/40 in either eye or a 2-line or more difference between each eye, even if in passing range (eg, 20/25 and 20/40).

- Distance visual acuity measurement for older children

  - Test with Snellen letters at 10 feet.

  - Refer if less than 20/30 or a 2-line or more difference between each eye even if in passing range.

- Optic nerve health and retinal vessels

  - Use direct ophthalmoscopy for cooperative children.

- Color vision deficiencies

  - Consider the Ishihara Test to assess color vision.

  - Color vision deficiencies are common in boys (5%–8%) but the value of screening is debated.

If possible, consider testing within a quiet room and not in a heavily trafficked hallway.

What Should You Do With an Abnormal Result?

Refer all children with an abnormal screening result to a pediatric ophthalmologist or an eye care specialist appropriately trained to treat pediatric patients. Some optometrists offer vision therapy, based on eye exercises, for a number of different vision problems, including strabismus. The benefit of vision therapy is unclear. Insurance often does not cover vision therapy.

Refer children at high risk regardless of screening results.

Some children who have vision problems will appear to be uncooperative with testing. When in doubt, refer.

Some children will not receive follow-up care because some parents do not understand the benefits of early detection. Explain these benefits to all families at the time of referral.

Some children do not have coverage for the treatment of refractive errors. Become aware of local available resources (eg, Lions Club). Medicaid provides vision coverage, including corrective lenses.

What Results Should You Document?

Document vision in the medical record and refer as appropriate.

These *CPT* codes were specifically developed to report vision screening tests. Most health plans provide benefit coverage for vision screening; however, payment for vision screening may be inappropriately bundled with the health supervision visit.

Resources

Article

American Academy of Pediatrics Committee on Practice and Ambulatory Medicine, Section on Ophthalmology; American Association of Certified Orthoptists; American Association for Pediatric Ophthalmology and Strabismus; American Academy of Ophthalmology. Eye examination in infants, children, and young adults by pediatricians. *Pediatrics*. 2003;111:902–907

CPT and *ICD-9-CM* Codes	
360.44	Leukocoria
366.0	Infantile, juvenile, and presenile cataract
743.2	Congenital glaucoma
743.61	Congenital ptosis
743.3	Congenital cataract and lens anomalies
368.0	Amblyopia
378	Strabismus and other disorders of binocular eye movements
367.0	Hyperopia
367.1	Myopia
368.5	Color vision deficiencies
99173	Screening tests of visual acuity, quantitative, bilateral
99174	Ocular photoscreening with interpretation and report, bilateral

The American Academy of Pediatrics publishes a complete line of coding publications, including an annual edition of *Coding for Pediatrics*. For more information on these excellent resources, visit the American Academy of Pediatrics Online Bookstore at **www.aap.org/bookstore/.**

Tool

- HOTV chart
- Lea chart (heart, house, circle, square)
- Snellen numbers
- Random Dot E stereotest

ANTICIPATORY GUIDANCE

The anticipatory guidance component of every Bright Futures visit gives the health care professional, parents, and the child or adolescent a chance to ask questions and discuss issues of concern. This guidance is organized around 5 priority areas, and specific questions and discussion points are provided for the health care professional. Health care professionals are encouraged to adapt and enhance these questions and discussion points to meet the specific needs of their families and communities.

The chapters in this section of the book focus on topics of public health importance, in which active discussion and guidance can make a positive impact in the lives of families. For example, the **Motivational Interviewing** chapter provides a framework to help health care professionals talk to patients and families about behavior change, a subject that is central to all the topics in this section of the book.

ANTICIPATORY GUIDANCE

JOEL BASS, MD

BICYCLE HELMETS

Why Is It Important to Include Bicycle Helmets in Anticipatory Guidance?

Many children and youth love to bicycle but they don't always wear a helmet. Bicycling is a popular recreational activity in the United States, particularly among children. It is estimated that 33 million children ride bicycles for nearly 10 billion hours each year.

Unfortunately, only 25% of children use helmets all or most of the time while cycling.[1]

Bicycle-related injuries are common. Every year, about 450,000 children are treated in emergency departments for bicycle-related injuries. Of the injuries, 153,000 are for head injuries. These head injuries are often very serious and account for most bicycle-related deaths.

Many of the nonfatal injuries also are of great consequence, often producing lifelong disability associated with brain damage.[2]

Bicycle helmets protect children. It is well established that bicycle helmets are effective in preventing head injuries associated with bicycling. Overall, helmets decrease the risk of head and brain injury by about 80%.[3] The risk of facial injuries to the upper and mid face is reduced by 65%.[3]

Counseling and safety programs can increase helmet use. Although not specific to bicycle helmet counseling, injury prevention counseling of parents of young children in the primary care setting has been shown to result in enhanced educational and behavioral outcomes. In some cases, it has resulted in decreased injuries.[4]

Effective programs directed specifically at increasing the use of bicycle helmets in children have leveraged the synergy of legislation, community-based initiatives, and economic incentives.[1] One report, which also included reinforcing community initiatives with advice from pediatric practices, resulted in a significant increase in helmet use.[5]

How Should You Provide Anticipatory Guidance About Bicycle Helmets?

Urge parents to

- Check that the helmet meets the bicycle safety standards of the Consumer Product Safety Commission.

- Fit the helmet squarely on top of the child's head, covering the forehead. Be certain that it does not move around on the head or slide down. Adjust the chin strap to a snug fit.

- Be certain that the child wears the helmet every time he or she rides the bike.

- Serve as a model for the child. Parents also should always wear a helmet when bicycle riding.

Use materials from the American Academy of Pediatrics (AAP) Injury Prevention Program (TIPP) to enhance your counseling. The TIPP sheets "About Bicycle Helmets" and "Tips for Getting Your Children to Wear Bicycle Helmets" have additional educational points.

Consider performing an actual assessment of the helmet in your office. It can provide further reinforcement and education about bicycle helmets.[6]

ANTICIPATORY GUIDANCE

161

What Anticipatory Guidance Should You Provide if You Encounter Resistance to Helmet Use?

Give parents who do not require their children to use a helmet extensive information about the risks of bicycle-related head injuries, including the TIPP sheets and details of state or local legislation or regulations.

Whenever available, provide discount coupons for approved helmets. If your community has an active helmet program, they may provide access to free helmets under certain circumstances.

Children who answer that they do not use a bicycle helmet should be given information appropriate to their age and cognitive level on the need for helmets. Materials for children from ongoing state or local community programs also may be available.

What Results Should You Document?

Documentation of counseling efforts is always recommended. The physician copies of the Framingham Safety Surveys also are useful for documentation and to identify patients who would benefit from reviewing the issue of helmet use at subsequent visits.

CPT and ICD-9-CM Codes	
99401	Preventive medicine counseling or risk factor reduction intervention(s) provided to an individual; approximately 15 minutes.

The American Academy of Pediatrics publishes a complete line of coding publications, including an annual edition of *Coding for Pediatrics*. For more information on these excellent resources, visit the American Academy of Pediatrics Online Bookstore at **www.aap.org/bookstore/**.

Resources

Tools

The AAP TIPP Program has injury prevention counseling questionnaires, including the Framingham Safety Survey: From 5 to 9 Years and from 10 to 12 Years. This survey covers the issue of bicycle helmet use. The 5 to 9 Years survey is completed by the parent and the 10 to 12 Years survey is completed by the child. Each survey includes a physician copy in which at-risk responses are easily identified.[7] This provides a useful, interactive method to counsel parents and children and also provides documentation of the counseling process.

Web Sites

American Academy of Pediatrics: http://www.aap.org/

Bicycle Helmet Safety Institute http://www.bhsi.org/index.htm

Centers for Disease Control and Prevention: http://www.cdc.gov/

Harborview Injury Prevention and Research Center: http://depts.washington.edu/hiprc/

References

1. Bicycle injury interventions: education background. Harborview Injury Prevention & Research Center Web Site. 2010. http://depts.washington.edu/hiprc/practices/topic/bicycles/helmeteduc.html

2. Injury-Control Recommendations: Bicycle Helmets. MMWR, 44(16), 325 (1995). available at: cdc.gov/.mmwr/preview/mmwrhtml/00036941.htm

3. Bicycle injury interventions: programs to increase helmet use. Harborview Injury Prevention & Research Center Web Site. 2010. http://depts.washington.edu/hiprc/practices/topic/bicycles/helmeteduc.html

4. Bass JL, Christoffel KK, Widome MW, et al. Childhood injury prevention counseling in primary care settings: a critical review of the literature. Pediatrics. 1993;92:544–550

5. Abularrage JJ, DeLuca AJ, Abularrage CJ. Effect of education and legislation on bicycle helmet use in a multiracial population. *Arch Pediatr Adolesc Med.* 1997;151:41–44

6. Parkinson GW, Hike KE. Bicycle helmet assessment during well visits reveals severe shortcomings in condition and fit. *Pediatrics.* 2003;112:320–323

7. American Academy of Pediatrics Committee and Section on Injury, Violence and Poison Prevention. TIPP: *A Guide to Safety Counseling in Office Practice.* Elk Grove Village, IL: American Academy of Pediatrics; 1994

VICTOR C. STRASBURGER, MD

CHILDREN, ADOLESCENTS, AND MEDIA

Why Is It Important to Include Media Usage in Anticipatory Guidance?

Children and teenagers spend more than 7 hours a day with a variety of different media.[1] Television predominates, with more than 4 hours a day of screen time, although viewing may now be via a computer or a cell phone screen instead of a TV set. Media use represents the *leading* leisure time activity for young people—they spend more time with media than they do in any other activity except sleeping. Increasingly, preteens and teens are using new technologies (social networking sites, cell phones) to communicate with each other; but there are documented risks to this as well, including bullying and displays of risky behaviors online and in text messages.[2–4]

Thousands of studies now attest to the power of the media to influence virtually every concern that pediatricians and parents have about the health and development of children and adolescents—sex, drugs, obesity, school achievement, bullying, eating disorders, and even attention-deficit disorder (ADD) and attention-deficit/hyperactivity disorder (ADHD).[5] The research has been well documented and summarized in a number of American Academy of Pediatrics (AAP) policy statements and in recent books.

Media violence. The impact of television in particular on aggressive behavior in young people has been documented since the early 1950s in more than 2,000 published studies. While media violence is not the leading cause of violence in society, it can be a significant factor. In addition, virtually everyone is *desensitized* by the violence they see on TV, movie, and video screens. American media specialize in portraying the notion of *justifiable violence* (eg, "good" guys versus "bad" guys). In the research literature, this is the single most powerful positive reinforcer for producing aggression. Bullying online and via text messaging is also an increasing concern.

Sex. Television shows for teenagers actually contain more sexual content than adults' shows, yet less than 10% of that content involves the discussion of risks or responsibilities involved in sexual relationships. In the absence of effective sex education at home or in schools, the media have arguably become the leading sex educator in the United States. Several longitudinal studies now link exposure to sexual content at a young age to earlier onset of sexual intercourse. In addition, up to 20% of teens have engaged in "sexting."[6]

Drugs. More than $20 billion a year is spent advertising legal drugs in the United States—$13 billion on cigarettes, $5 billion on alcohol, and $4 billion on prescription drugs. Numerous studies have found that advertising can be a potent influence on whether teenagers will start using cigarettes or alcohol. New research has found that witnessing smoking or drinking alcohol in movies may be the leading factor associated with adolescent onset of substance use.

Obesity. Dozens of studies have implicated media in the current worldwide epidemic of obesity; however, the mechanism is unclear. Young people see an estimated 10,000 food ads per year on TV, most of them for junk food or fast food. Screen time increases unhealthy snacking, may displace more active pursuits, and may interfere with healthy sleep habits.

Eating disorders. The impact of media on unhealthy body self-image, especially in young girls, has been well documented, especially in advertising and mainstream media. Two studies have linked media use with eating disorders.

Other health concerns. Several studies have linked media use with ADD, ADHD, and poorer school performance. In addition, half a dozen studies have found potential language delays in infants younger than 2 years exposed to TV or videos.

Prosocial media. While all of these potential health problems exist, clinicians also need to recognize the extraordinary power of the media to teach prosocial attitudes and behaviors like empathy, cooperation, tolerance, and even school readiness skills. Media have an amazing ability to teach—the only question is, what are children and teenagers learning from them?

Should You Screen for Media Usage?

Since they potentially influence numerous aspects of child and adolescent health, the media may represent the most important area of anticipatory guidance in well-child visits. One study has shown that a minute or two of office counseling about media violence and guns could reduce violence exposure for nearly 1 million children per year.[7] Given the sheer number of hours that children and teens spend with media, as well as the convincing research on health effects of the media, counseling is imperative. Parents are also looking for help, especially understanding and supervising computer use and social networking sites.

How Should You Screen for Media Usage?

To screen for media usage, clinicians should ask 2 questions about media use at health supervision visits:

(1) How much screen time per day does the child spend? and

(2) Is there a TV set or Internet connection in the child's bedroom?

The AAP Media Matters campaign developed a media history form for parents that can be filled out while waiting to see a clinician.

Because of the research findings, children or teens who are overweight or obese, have school problems, exhibit aggressive behavior, display sexual precociousness, or are depressed or suicidal should be asked specifically about how much screen time they spend and what programs, specifically, they are watching.

What Anticipatory Guidance Should You Provide Regarding Media Usage?

The AAP makes the following recommendations for advising parents:

- Limit total entertainment screen time to fewer than 2 hours per day.
- Avoid screen time for babies younger than 2 years.
- Encourage a careful selection of programs to view.
- Coview and discuss content with children and adolescents.
- Teach critical viewing skills.
- Limit and focus time spent with media. In particular, parents of young children and preteens should avoid exposing them to PG-13 and R-rated movies.
- Be good media role models—children often develop their media habits based on their parents' media behavior.
- Emphasize alternative activities.
- Create an "electronic media–free" environment in children's rooms.
- Avoid use of media as an electronic babysitter.
- Avoid watching TV during family meals.

What Results Should You Document?

Total amount of screen time per day and presence of a TV set or an Internet connection in the bedroom should be documented.

Resources

AAP Policy Statements

American Academy of Pediatrics Committee on Communications. Children, adolescents, and advertising. *Pediatrics*. 2006;118:2563–2569

American Academy of Pediatrics Committee on Public Education. Sexuality, contraception, and the media. *Pediatrics*. 2001;107:191–194

American Academy of Pediatrics Council on Communications and Media. Policy statement: media violence. *Pediatrics*. 2009;124:1495–1503

Books

Christakis DA, Zimmerman FJ. *The Elephant in the Living Room: Make Television Work for Your Kids*. New York, NY: Rodale Press; 2006

Strasburger VC, Wilson BJ, Jordan AB. *Children, Adolescents, and the Media*. 2nd ed. Thousand Oaks, CA: Sage; 2009

Web Sites

American Academy of Pediatrics: www.aap.org

Center on Media and Child Health: http://www.cmch.tv/ Online library of research articles.

Children's Health Topics: Internet & Media Use: http://www.aap.org/healthtopics/mediause.cfm

Common Sense Media: http://www.commonsensemedia.org/
Ratings and advice for parents on a variety of different media.

Council on Communications and Media blog: http://cocm.blogspot.com/

Kaiser Family Foundation: http://www.kff.org
Many content analyses and review articles on children and media.

Media history form: http://www.aap.org/advocacy/Media%20History%20Form.pdf

Advice for Parents

AAP: SafetyNet: Keep Your Children Safe Online: http://safetynet.aap.org/

References

1. Rideout V. *Generation M2: Media in the Lives of 8- to 18-Year-Olds*. Menlo Park, CA: Kaiser Family Foundation; 2010

2. Moreno M. Update on social networking sites. *Pediatr Ann*. In press

3. Moreno MA, Parks MR, Zimmerman FJ, Brito TE, Christakis DA. Display of health risk behaviors on MySpace by adolescents: prevalence and associations. *Arch Pediatr Adolesc Med*. 2009;163:27–34

4. Ybarra ML, Espelage DL, Mitchell KJ. The co-occurrence of Internet harassment and unwanted sexual solicitation victimization and perpetration: associations with psychosocial indicators. *J Adolesc Health*. 2007;41:S31–S41

5. Strasburger VC, Jordan AB, Donnerstein E. Health effects of media on children and adolescents. *Pediatrics*. 2010;125(4):756–767

6. National Campaign to Prevent Teen and Unplanned Pregnancy. *Sex and Tech*. Washington, DC: National Campaign to Prevent Teen and Unplanned Pregnancy; 2008

7. Barkin SL, Finch SA, Ip EH, et al. Is office-based counseling about media use, timeouts, and firearm storage effective? Results from a cluster-randomized, controlled trial. *Pediatrics*. 2008;122(1):e15–e25

STEPHEN COOK, MD

CARDIOMETABOLIC RISK OF OBESITY

Metabolic syndrome is a clustering constellation of metabolic and physiologic derangements that portend type 2 diabetes and premature cardiovascular disease. Although Bright Futures does not include screening recommendations for this syndrome, the American Academy of Pediatrics (AAP) has issued a recent policy statement regarding lipid screening and cardiovascular health in childhood, which includes blood pressure assessment. Anticipatory guidance to help children maintain normal blood lipids and blood pressure—2 key components involved in metabolic syndrome—is a crucial part of preventive services for children and adolescents.

What Is Metabolic Syndrome?

An individual is said to have metabolic syndrome if he or she meets 3 or more of the following 5 criteria:

- Age- and gender-specific elevated blood pressure (systolic blood pressure and/or diastolic blood pressure ≥90th percentile)

- Elevated waist circumference

- Elevated triglycerides

- Low high-density lipoprotein (HDL) cholesterol

- Elevated fasting glucose (≥100 mg/dL)

Although a recent paper from the American Heart Association suggested that using a specific definition or diagnostic criteria for children or adolescents is premature at this time.[1] The focus should be on excess adiposity or obesity; the cardiometabolic complications with excess weight; and the lifestyle factors of nutrition, physical activity, or tobacco use that elevate the risk for premature heart disease.

Why Is It Important to Include Metabolic Syndrome in Anticipatory Guidance?

The components of metabolic syndrome increase the risk of type 2 diabetes and premature cardiovascular disease among obese children.[2] The syndrome itself should not be a focus on diagnosis or treatment, but rather serve as a reminder to consider screening for these components as well as other metabolic abnormalities among obese youth.[1]

Overweight and obesity lead to the development of cardiometabolic abnormalities, like those described by the metabolic syndrome, as well as polycystic ovary syndrome (PCOS), sleep apnea, and nonalcoholic fatty liver disease (NAFLD). Obese children and adolescents are at increased risk for type 2 diabetes mellitus and premature cardiovascular disease in early adulthood.[3,4] A 3-year follow-up of 33 children with abnormal oral glucose tolerance test (OGTT) found 24% developed type 2 diabetes mellitus. Those who developed type 2 diabetes had persistent weight gain, were more overweight, and were African American.[5] Obese children with NAFLD, compared to matched obese youth without NAFLD, had 3 times the risk of having a metabolic syndrome clustering of risk factors.[6] Thus when clinicians detect features of the metabolic syndrome in obese youth, we must be aware of the risk of NAFLD.

Autopsy studies show that raised atheromatous plaques were present as early as 8 years of age. Further, overweight teens and young adults had more fatty streaks and larger cholesterol plaques than their normal-weight peers, and the severity of these lesions increased with each additional cardiometabolic abnormality.[7–9]

The US Preventive Services Task Force (USPSTF) found good evidence that overweight youth ages 8 years and older are at elevated risk for medical complications of their weight and at greatly elevated risk of becoming obese adults.[10] In early 2010, the USPSTF recommended that clinicians screen children 6 years of age and older for obesity and offer them or refer them to intensive counseling and behavioral interventions to promote improvements in weight status. (Grade B recommendation). These programs were described as comprehensive moderate- to high-intensity programs that include dietary, physical activity, and behavioral counseling components. These typically involved at least 25 hours of contact with the child and/or the family over a 6-month period.[11]

Cardiometabolic derangements among obese subjects is related to lifestyle behaviors, including diet and physical activity. Longitudinal studies show that these factors cluster together over time, especially among teens who demonstrate poor lifestyle behaviors. The Young Finns study showed a cluster of similar cardiovascular risk factors either remained abnormal or got worse over time if teens consumed excess calories, fat, and saturated fat; started or continued to smoke; or decreased their level of exercise.[12–14]

How Should You Determine Whether a Child Is at Risk for Cardiometabolic Abnormalities of Excess Weight?

Measure Body Mass Index (BMI)

Measure weight and height beginning at age 2 and calculate and plot BMI for age and gender at *all* health supervision visits. Details on measurement may be found in the "Assessing Growth and Nutrition" chapter.

Measure Blood Pressure

Measure blood pressure at *all* health supervision visits beginning with the 3-year visit. Confirm all blood pressure readings against updated blood pressure guidelines for children, and repeat abnormal measurements manually with an appropriate-sized cuff. Details on measurement may be found in the "Blood Pressure" chapter.

Screen for Dyslipidemias

The AAP policy statement, "Lipid Screening and Cardiovascular Health in Children,"[15] suggests that targeted screening for cholesterol, low-density lipoprotein (LDL) cholesterol, HDL cholesterol, and triglycerides with a fasting lipid panel now be considered for children with

- A positive family history of premature cardiovascular disease (myocardial infarct or stroke in men younger than 55 or women younger than 60, or with dyslipidemia)

- Family history of premature cardiovascular disease or dyslipidemia unknown

- Obesity, hypertension, or diabetes

An alternative to using single generic cut points to identify abnormalities in cholesterol, LDL cholesterol, HDL cholesterol, and triglycerides for boys and girls, now age- and gender-specific cut points for each of these have been developed.[16] (See Table 1.)

Although no management guidelines exist for metabolic syndrome specifically, any of these cardiometabolic complications of obesity should first be addressed with lifestyle changes. Weight loss goal recommendations and lifestyle changes rely on modification of diet and activity. Although difficult to make changes without ongoing reinforcement, counseling or referral to experienced weight loss providers should occur, and the pediatrician should be aware of youth activity programs in the area. Also, consider repeating blood tests in 3 to 6 months to confirm any abnormal results and consider additional screening if warranted by history or physical examination. Repeat blood tests every 6 to 12 months if weight maintenance or loss is not occurring.

Screen for Insulin Resistance and Type 2 Diabetes

Because insulin resistant is a key factor in this syndrome; overweight patients may need to be screened for type 2 diabetes. Screening may occur with a fasting glucose. If fasting blood glucose is greater than 100, an OGTT should be performed or the fasting glucose should be repeated in 3 months. Metabolic syndrome has been shown to

Table 1. Lipid and Lipoprotein in Distribution in Subjects Aged 5 to 18 Years

	Males			Females		
	5–9 y	10–14 y	15–18 y	5–9 y	10–14 y	15–18 y
Total Cholesterol (mg/dl)						
50th	164	160	153	127	161	159
75th	184	182	174	186	181	180
90th	203	203	197	207	202	202
95th	216	217	212	221	215	216
Triglycerides						
50th	62	66	72	67	76	72
75th	83	92	101	90	102	99
90th	114	128	143	123	141	137
95th	142	160	178	151	175	171
LDL Cholesterol						
50th	91	89	87	95	92	89
75th	109	108	106	114	111	108
90th	127	128	126	134	130	128
95th	120	141	139	147	143	140
HDL Cholesterol						
5th	38	34	31	35	35	35
10th	41	37	34	39	38	38
25th	48	43	39	45	44	44
50th	55	51	46	53	51	52

Source: Adapted from Tables IIB, IIIB, IVB, VB from Cook et al.[16]

progress to type 2 diabetes in very obese adolescents, and obese youth with impaired glucose tolerance are more likely to go on to develop type 2 diabetes sooner than are obese teens with the syndrome without impaired glucose tolerance.[17]

Acanthosis nigricans (Figure 1) with skin tags are a sign of insulin resistance. The presence of acanthosis nigricans actually correlates more closely with level of obesity and is therefore very common among obese adolescents with or without insulin resistance.

Acanthosis nigricans is considered a risk factor for screening for type 2 diabetes as part of the recommendations of the American Diabetes Association and the AAP.

Figure 1. Acanthosis nigricans

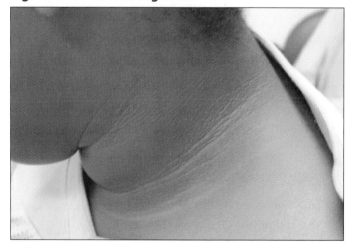

Figure 2. Visceral and subcutaneous fat on cross-section

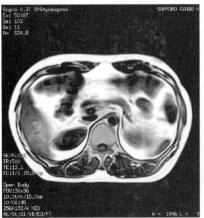
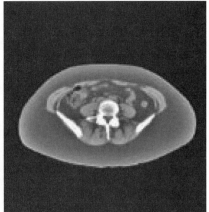
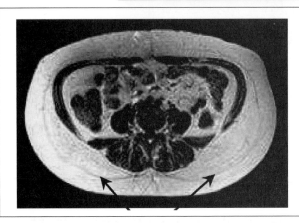
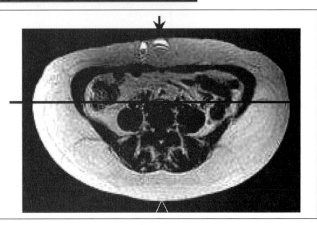

Measure Waist Circumference

Visceral adipose tissue (Figure 2) is fat tissue found in the intra-abdominal cavity and is an important component of excess central fat tissue because it has been shown to have different metabolic properties than subcutaneous fat. Excess visceral fat is associated with increased insulin resistance and dyslipidemia related to free fatty acid turnover.

Consider measuring waist circumference in children and adolescents who are overweight but not obese (BMI below the 95th percentile) but whom you think may have excess central fat.[10,18,19] To measure waist circumference (Figure 3)

- Locate the upper hip bone and the iliac crest.

- Place a measuring tape in the horizontal plane around the abdomen at the level of the iliac crest. Ensure that the tape is snug but does not compress the skin and is parallel to the floor.

- Take the measurement at the end of a normal expiration.

Figure 3. Measuring waist circumference.[a]

To measure waist circumference, locate the upper hip bone and the top of the right iliac crest. Place a measuring tape in a horizontal plane around the abdomen at the level of the iliac crest. Before reading the tape measure, ensure that the tape is snug, but does not compress the skin, and is parallel to the floor. The measurement is made at the end of a normal expiration.

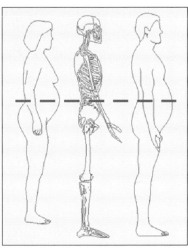

Measuring-Tape Position for Waist (Abdominal) Circumference in Adults

[a]Source: National Institutes of Health. Clinical guidelines on the identification, evaluation, and treatment of overweight and obesity in adults—the evidence report. National Institutes of Health. *Obes Res.* 1998;6(suppl 2):51S–209S.

For children younger than 18, values above the 90th percentile reflect an excess of central adipose tissue for age and sex (Table 2).

For adolescents older than 18, males with waist circumference greater than 40 inches (>102 cm) or females with waist circumferences greater than 35 inches (>88 cm) exceed the criteria for the adult definition of metabolic syndrome (Table 2). The high normal values from smoothed growth curves are meant to transition measures of excess abdominal fat during adolescence to abdominal obesity in adulthood at age 18.[16]

Table 2. Waist Circumference (cm) Cutoffs for Males and Females for > 50th and > 90th and for Age/Gender Specific High-Normal Values That Correlate to Adult Cut Offs

Age	Males			Females		
	50th	90th	High–Normal 91st	50th	90th	High–Normal 75th
2	48	53	53	48	53	50
3	50	55	55	50	56	53
4	52	58	58	52	59	55
5	53	61	61	53	61	57
6	55	64	65	55	64	59
7	57	69	69	57	69	62
8	60	73	74	60	73	66
9	63	78	79	63	78	69
10	65	83	83	66	83	73
11	68	87	87	70	87	78
12	71	91	91	73	91	81
13	73	94	95	75	94	83
14	75	96	97	76	96	85
15	77	98	99	77	97	86
16	79	100	100	78	98	87
17	80	101	101	79	99	87
18	81	101	102	79	100	88
Adult			102 cm			88 cm

The cut-off for abdominal obesity for men is 102 cm and for women it is 88 cm according to the NCEP guidelines. The 91st percentile curve for boys and the 75th percentile curves line for girls represent a smooth growth curve line that transitions into the respective adult cut-off values for abdominal obesity.

Source: Adapted from Table IB from Cook et al.[16]

What Should You Do With an Abnormal Result?

Follow Up

Abnormal laboratory values from a single point are not diagnostic for any obesity comorbidity like hypertension or hypercholesterolemia. Follow up with the patient and family relatively soon after these results come in.

Inform the patient and family of the abnormal results.

- Assess and assist patients with weight maintenance or weight loss efforts.
- Guide further or additional screening for cardio-metabolic complications of obesity such as NAFLD or PLOS.

Provide Treatment and Counseling

Overweight and Obesity

Weight loss is the primary target for treating cardio-metabolic abnormalities of obesity. Include family members when behavioral change for weight loss is the goal.[4,18] This is especially true for this cardiometabolic clustering for 2 reasons.

- The clustering of abnormalities in metabolic syndrome occurs in adults and their offspring. Parents with the syndrome are very likely to have children with the syndrome.[20,21] If one or both parents are overweight, they will benefit from behavior changes that lead to weight loss in the child.
- Parent behavior change and weight loss are some of the strongest predictors of child weight loss.[22]

A general low-calorie diet with reduced total fat, as recommended by National Institutes of Health guidelines and the American Heart Association, will benefit the whole family.[4,23] The child and parents should partner with behavior changes around food and avoid so-called fad diets.

Regular daily exercise, preferably 60 minutes of moderate to vigorous physical activity, is recommended. To help the family achieve their weight loss and physical activity goals, counsel the family to also decrease sedentary behavior, such as television viewing and other forms of screen time, to less than 2 hours per day.[4]

The "Weight Maintenance and Weight Loss" chapter provides further details on overweight and obesity assessment and anticipatory guidance.

Cardiovascular Risk Factors

The AAP policy statement, "Lipid Screening and Cardiovascular Health in Children,"[15] suggests the use of statins as a first-line treatment for children as young as 8 years with dyslipidemia, defined as abnormalities in total cholesterol, LDL, HDL, and trigycerides, as described previously.

Type 2 Diabetes

Counsel patients and families on signs and symptoms of diabetes, especially in severely obese youth with a family history of type 2 diabetes.

Although your comfort level and regional practice patterns should dictate care, for those children and youth with impaired fasting glucose or abnormal glucose tolerance tests, consider referral to an endocrinologist (pediatric or adult) or to a specialist comfortable in the management of type 2 diabetes in youth. If the child cannot be seen by the specialist for a considerable time, strongly consider instructing the family about in-home glucose monitoring and starting an insulin-sensitizing agent such as metformin.

Sleep Abnormalities

This syndrome is associated with obstructive sleep apnea syndrome (OSAS). Obese subjects with snoring should be referred for diagnostic testing (polysomnography) to quantify the degree of OSAS as well as guide options for therapy.[24]

Liver Problems

Metabolic syndrome and insulin resistance are associated with nonalcoholic fatty liver disease, which can progress to nonalcoholic steatohepatitis (NASH), also called fatty liver. Liver enzyme testing is warranted to test for this condition.

Weight loss with diet and exercise is recommended as the first-line therapy for NASH, but clinical trials are ongoing examining the benefit of antioxidant supplements to improve the inflammatory process in the liver.

Menstrual Irregularities

Females with metabolic syndrome and irregular periods may have PCOS. Consider testing for elevated insulin and testosterone (free or total) levels if a female patient with metabolic syndrome continues to have irregular menstrual cycles. Consider a referral to an endocrinologist (pediatric or adult) or an obstetrician/gynecologist comfortable in the management of PCOS.

What Results Should We Document?

Document weight at all visits. Height measurements can be limited to every 6 months for BMI calculation.

Measure and record blood pressure at all visits beginning with the 3-year visit. Measure blood pressure of obese adolescents with an appropriate-sized cuff and technique.

At all visits, track and record weight change, blood pressure change, and goals for both weight and blood pressure.

Resources

American Diabetes Association. Type 2 diabetes in children and adolescents. *Pediatrics.* 2000;105:671–680

Krebs NF, Jacobson MS; American Academy of Pediatrics Committee on Nutrition. Prevention of pediatric overweight and obesity. *Pediatrics.* 2003;112(2):424–430

Obesity in Adolescence: Part 1
Sandra Hassink, *Adolescent Health Update,* Vol 21, No. 1 October 2008. p 1-9

Obesity in Adolescence, Part 2: Cardiometabolic Risks
Megan Gabel and Stephen Cook, Adolescent Health Update, Vol 21, No. 2 February 2009. p 1-9

ICD-9-CM Codes

277.7	Syndrome X; dysmetabolic syndrome This code can only be used if *ICD-9-CM* codes for overweight, obesity, or morbid obesity are used first.
278.00	Overweight/obesity
278.01	Morbid obesity

Consider including related diagnostic codes for individual components of the syndrome (elevated blood pressure without hypertension, impaired fasting glucose, hyperinsulinemia, dyslipidemia, impaired glucose tolerance). This approach is strongly advised if the patient only has one or two components of the syndrome and thus does not qualify for third-party payer coverage for metabolic syndrome.

251.1	Hyperinsulinism (ectopic, functional, organic; excludes hypoglycemia)
272.4	Dyslipidemia
401.9	Hypertension (unspecified)
701.2	Acanthosis nigricans
790.21	Impaired fasting glucose
790.22	Impaired glucose tolerance

Additionally, the use of the *CPT* code set **99401–99404**—preventive medicine counseling/risk-factor reduction—may also be relevant when providing guidance and counseling on risk-factor reduction.

99401	Preventive medicine counseling and/or risk-factor reduction intervention(s) provided to an individual (separate procedure); approximately 15 minutes
99402	approximately 30 minutes
99403	approximately 45 minutes
99404	approximately 60 minutes

For more information on reporting these codes, see AAP *Coding for Pediatrics 2010* (pages 62–63).

The American Academy of Pediatrics publishes a complete line of coding publications, including an annual edition of *Coding for Pediatrics*. For more information on these excellent resources, visit the American Academy of Pediatrics Online Bookstore at **www.aap.org/bookstore/**.

References

1. Steinberger J, Daniels SR, Eckel RH, et al. Progress and challenges in metabolic syndrome in children and adolescents: A scientific statement from the American Heart Association Atherosclerosis, Hypertension, and Obesity in the Young Committee of the Council on Cardiovascular Disease in the Young; Council on Cardiovascular Nursing; and Council on Nutrition, Physical Activity, and Metabolism. *Circulation*. 2009;119:628–647

2. Morrison J, Friedman L, Gray-McGuire C. Metabolic syndrome in childhood predicts adult cardiovascular disease 25 years later: the Princeton Lipid Research Clinics follow-up study. *Pediatrics*, 2007;120: 340–345

3. Cook S, Weitzman M, Auinger P, Nguyen M, Dietz WH. Prevalence of a metabolic syndrome phenotype in adolescents: findings from the Third National Health and Nutrition Examination Survey, 1988–1994. *Arch Of Pediatr Adolesc Med*. 2003;157:821–827

4. Daniels SR, Arnett DK, Eckel RH, et al. Overweight in children and adolescents: pathophysiology, consequences, prevention, and treatment. *Circulation*. 2005;111(15):1999–2012

5. Matyka K. Type 2 diabetes in childhood: epidemiological and clinical aspects. *Br Med Bull*. 2008;86(1):59–75

6. Schwimmer JB, Pardee PE, Lavine JE, Blumkin AK, Cook S. Cardiovascular risk factors and the metabolic syndrome in pediatric nonalcoholic fatty liver disease. *Circulation*. 2008;118:277–283

7. Berenson GS, Srinivasan SR, Bao W, Newman WP, Tracy RE, Wattigney WA. Association between multiple cardiovascular risk factors and atherosclerosis in children and young adults. The Bogalusa Heart Study. *N Engl J Med*. 1998;338(23):1650–1656

8. McGill HC Jr, McMahan CA, Herderick EE, et al. Obesity accelerates the progression of coronary atherosclerosis in young men. *Circulation*. 2002;105(23):2712–2718

9. Raitakari OT, Juonala M, Kahonen M, et al. Cardiovascular risk factors in childhood and carotid artery intima-media thickness in adulthood: the Cardiovascular Risk in Young Finns Study. *JAMA*. 2003;290(17):2277–2283

10. US Preventive Services Task Force. Screening and interventions for overweight in children and adolescents: recommendation statement. *Pediatrics*. 2005;116:205–209

11. US Preventive Services Task Force. Screening for obesity in children and adolescents: US Preventive Services Task Force recommendation statement. *Pediatrics*. 2010;125:361–367

12. Raitakari OT, Leino M, Rakkonen K, et al. Clustering of risk habits in young adults. The Cardiovascular Risk in Young Finns Study. *Am J Epidemiol*. 1995;142(1):36–44

13. Katzmarzyk PT, Perusse L, Malina RM, Bergeron J, Despres JP, Bouchard C. Stability of indicators of the metabolic syndrome from childhood and adolescence to young adulthood: the Quebec Family Study. *J Clin Epidemiol*. 2001;54:190–195

14. Juonala M, Viikari JS, Hutri-Kahonen N, et al. The 21-year follow-up of the Cardiovascular Risk in Young Finns Study: risk factor levels, secular trends and east-west difference. *J Intern Med.* 2004;255:457–468

15. Daniels S, Greer F; American Academy of Pediatrics Committee on Nutrition. Lipid screening and cardiovascular health in childhood. *Pediatrics.* 2008;122(1):198–208

16. Cook S, Auinger P, Huang TT. Growth curves for cardiometabolic risk factors in children and adolescents. *J Pediatr.* 2009;155:e15–e26

17. Weiss R, Taksali SE, Tamborlane WV, Burgert T, Savoye M, Caprio S. Predictors of changes in glucose tolerance status in obese youth. *Diabetes Care.* 2005;28:902–909

18. Barlow SE, Dietz WH. Obesity evaluation and treatment: Expert Committee recommendations. The Maternal and Child Health Bureau, Health Resources and Services Administration and the Department of Health and Human Services. *Pediatrics.* 1998;102(3):e29

19. National High Blood Pressure Education Program Working Group on High Blood Pressure in Children and Adolescents. The fourth report on the diagnosis, evaluation, and treatment of high blood pressure in children and adolescents. *Pediatrics.* 2004;114:555–576

20. Pankow JS, Jacobs DR, Steinberger J, Moran A, Sinaiko AR. Insulin resistance and cardiovascular disease risk factors in children of parents with the insulin resistance (metabolic) syndrome. *Diabetes Care.* 2004;27:775–780

21. Chen W, Srinivasan SR, Elkasabany A, Berenson GS. The association of cardiovascular risk factor clustering related to insulin resistance syndrome (syndrome X) between young parents and their offspring: the Bogalusa Heart Study. *Atherosclerosis.* 1999;145(1):197–205

22. Wrotniak BH, Epstein LH, Paluch RA, Roemmich JN. Parent weight change as a predictor of child weight change in family-based behavioral obesity treatment. *Arch Pediatr Adolesc Med.* 2004;158:342–347

23. American Heart Association; Gidding SS, Dennison BA, et al. Dietary recommendations for children and adolescents: a guide for practitioners. *Pediatrics.* 2006;117:544–559

24. American Academy of Pediatrics Section on Pediatric Pulmonology, Subcommittee on Obstructive Sleep Apnea Syndrome. Clinical practice guideline: diagnosis and management of childhood obstructive sleep apnea syndrome. *Pediatrics.* 2002;109:704–712

ROBERT P. SCHWARTZ, MD

MOTIVATIONAL INTERVIEWING

Motivational interviewing (MI) is a shared decision-making strategy for enhancing a patient's motivation to make a behavior change—for example, in weight, tobacco, or safety counseling. It is a particularly helpful method in addressing resistance to change because it helps you create an alliance with the patient irrespective of his or her willingness to make a change. Although MI is not specifically described in Bright Futures, these methods are quite effective in providing many types of anticipatory guidance where a change is needed.

What Is Motivational Interviewing?

Motivational interviewing is a patient-centered guiding method for enhancing motivation to change.[1,2] Ambivalence is a stage in the normal process of change, and must be resolved for change to occur.[1] Motivational interviewing can be effective for those who are initially ambivalent about making behavior changes because it allows the person to explore and resolve their ambivalence.[1,2]

Motivational interviewing is a collaborative process of decision-making. Its style is empathetic, nonjudgmental, supportive, and nonconfrontational.[1,3] It acknowledges that behavior change is driven by motivation, not information. Motivation to change occurs when a person perceives a discrepancy or conflict between current behavior and important life goals, such as being healthy.[1,3] The reasons for behavior change arise from the patient's own goals or values, and it is up to the patient to find solutions to the problem.[1]

Why Is It Important to Use Motivational Interviewing in Anticipatory Guidance?

Physicians have been trained to provide information, but not how to help patients change their behavior. Pediatricians often lack confidence in their motivational and behavioral counseling skills. Training in MI may

improve your self-confidence in counseling skills and your efficacy in helping patients change behavior.

Motivational interviewing works. Randomized controlled trials have demonstrated the efficacy of MI in treating alcohol and substance abuse problems.[4–8]

Motivational interviewing also is being used to address other health behaviors, such as eating, smoking, physical activity, and adherence with treatment regimens.[3–5,7,9,10, 11]

Motivational interviewing may be useful with adolescents. Because of its lack of authoritarian style and avoidance of confrontation, MI may be effective in counseling adolescents.[5,6]

How Do You Do Motivational Interviewing?

The acronym **OARES** summarizes the key components of MI.[1]

- Ask **O**pen-ended questions.

  ▶ This type of question uses the patient's own words, is not biased or judgmental, and cannot be answered by a simple "yes" or "no." For example, instead of asking, "Are you feeling OK?" you might restate the question as, "Help me understand how you feel."

- **A**ffirm what your patient says.

  ▷ Affirmations are statements that recognize your patient's strengths and efforts. Example: "You are really connected to your family and friends."

- Use **R**eflective listening.

  ▷ This type of listening allows you to clarify the meaning and feeling of what your patient says. Examples: "It sounds like you are not happy in the relationship with your boyfriend." "You feel like nobody understands you."

- **E**licit self-motivational statements or "change talk."

  ▷ A person's belief in his or her ability to change is a good predictor of success. The first step in affirming this belief and to elicit "change talk" is to ask the patient about their level of "importance and confidence" in making a behavior change using the following scale.[1,3]

Importance and Confidence Scale

IMPORTANCE

On a scale of 0 to 10, with 10 being very important, how important is it for you to change?

0	1	2	3	4	5	6	7	8	9	10
Not at all				Somewhat					Very	

CONFIDENCE

On a scale of 0 to 10, with 10 being very confident, how confident are you that you can change?

0	1	2	3	4	5	6	7	8	9	10
Not at all				Somewhat					Very	

Follow this "importance and confidence" questions scale with 2 probes: "You chose (STATE NUMBER). Why didn't you choose a lower number?" This question elicits arguments for change by the patient. Then ask, "What would it take to get you to a higher number?" This identifies barriers.[3]

- **S**ummarize.

  ▷ At the end, summarize your conversation and decisions. This links together and reinforces what your patient has stated.

The acronym **FRAMES** is a brief adaptation of MI.[5,6]

- Provide **F**eedback on the risks and consequences of the behavior.

- Emphasize the patient's personal **R**esponsibility to change or not to change. "It's up to you."

- Provide **A**dvice—your professional opinion and recommendation.

- Offer **M**enus. You provide a menu of strategies, not a single solution. The patient selects the approach that seems best for him or her.

- Show **E**mpathy. A positive, caring manner will foster rapport.

- Encourage **S**elf-efficacy. Encourage positive "change talk" and support your patient in believing that he or she can change the behavior.

Continued resistance may indicate that you misjudged your patient's readiness or motivation to change.[12] Be empathetic and use reflective listening. You could respond by saying, "It sounds like this may not be the right time for you to make a change. Perhaps you are concerned about something else."

What Results Should You Document?

Document topics (behaviors) discussed, the patient's level of importance and confidence in making change, plans for follow-up, and time spent counseling.

Some insurance plans cover OTC products. Pharmacotherapies include

- Over-the-counter products, including nicotine gum, patch, lozenge. Be sure to read the directions for use. Using combinations of NRTs is recommended by the Tobacco Treatment Guideline to improve quit rates; however, combination use is considered off-label. Examples include use of the patch all day and chewing gum or using a lozenge when experiencing a craving. Most persons who report failure of these products as an aid to quitting used the product incorrectly, usually by not using the product as frequently as recommended.

- Prescription NRTs, including nicotine inhaler and nasal spray. Some incidence of addiction to these products has occurred. Prescription NRTs are typically covered by insurance plans.

- Other prescriptions that are non-nicotine include the selective serotonin reuptake inhibitor, bupropion, or the selective nicotinic modulator, varenicline.

  - Bupropion (Zyban). Reduces cravings and is prescription only. Begin using 7 to 14 days before quit date and continue for 12 or more weeks after quitting. Use may be combined with NRT products.

  - Varenicline (Chantix). Prescription only, a selective nicotinic receptor modulator. May be more effective than bupropion. Also used for 12 or more weeks. Do not combine with NRT products because of risk of nausea.

Adolescent Tobacco Users

Evidence is mixed on adolescent-specific approaches. The same techniques for cessation should be used with adolescents that you would use with adults, tailored to the adolescent.

How Should You Screen and Counsel for Tobacco Use Cessation?

Use the AAR or "5 As" Approach[3]

There are 2 recommended approaches to tobacco use cessation in the pediatric office setting. At a minimum, with parents as well as youth, ASK about tobacco use and tobacco smoke exposure, ADVISE to quit, and REFER for assistance to local resources or quit lines.

More effective, but more time consuming, are the 5 As.

- Ask
  - Obtain an applicable history from all patients and families.
  - Ask about current and past tobacco use, tobacco smoke exposure, and tobacco use before and during pregnancy. Some 70% of women who quit smoking during pregnancy will relapse in the first year of their baby's life.

- Advise
  - Look for "teachable moments."
  - Personalize the health risks of tobacco use.
  - Use clear, strong, personalized messages: "Smoking is harmful for you (and your child). Would you like to quit?" "How can I help you?"

- Assess
  - Determine whether the patient or parent is willing to make a behavior change.
  - Establish whether he or she is willing to try to quit tobacco use at this time.

- Assist
  - Provide information about tobacco use cessation to all tobacco users.
  - Strongly urge 100% smoke-free (and tobacco-free) home and car.
  - Help patients and parents set realistic and specific goals.
    - "Quit" date
    - "Smoke-free home and car" date
  - Help patients and parents prepare.
    - Get support.
    - Anticipate challenges.
    - Practice problem-solving.
    - Provide information about pharmacotherapy and cessation resources.

- Provide supplemental materials.

- Refer to telephone quit lines—preferably with "active" fax referral process that can be initiated in the medical office. Many quit lines will call the client directly, rather than having the smoker make the initiative to call by themselves. Many states have fax referral forms for medical practitioners to use. The United States universal quit line number is 1-800-QUIT NOW. This will refer directly to the state from which the phone call is initiated.

- Arrange Follow-up.

  ▸ Plan to follow up on any behavioral commitments that your patient makes.

  ▸ Schedule follow-up in person or by telephone soon after an important date, such as a quit date or anniversary.

Anticipate With Younger Patients

Anticipating is sometimes called the "sixth A." Discuss tobacco use with preteens and teens during health supervision visits. Include tobacco use with discussions of other risk behaviors, including alcohol, substance abuse, and sexual activity.

Be Prepared for the Unwilling and Not Ready

For the unwilling/not ready

The "5 Rs"

Relevance
- Discuss with the family and/or patient why quitting is particularly relevant to them, being as concrete as possible.

Risks
- Encourage the patient to identify the risks of tobacco use, highlighting the risks that are particularly salient to the patient.

Rewards
- Encourage the patient to identify the benefits of tobacco use, highlighting the benefits that are particularly salient to the patient.

CPT and ICD-9-CM Codes

305.1	Tobacco use disorder
V15.89	Other specified personal history presenting hazards to health (secondhand smoke exposure)
989.84	Toxic effects of tobacco—Use when the pediatrician documents that a child's illness is directly worsened or exacerbated by exposure to tobacco smoke.
E869.4	Secondhand tobacco smoke. This E-code was created to identify nonsmokers who have been exposed to tobacco smoke. This cannot be used as a principal diagnosis, but may be used when the tobacco smoke exposure is the external cause of the patient's condition.
99406	Smoking and tobacco use cessation counseling visit, intermediate, greater than 3 minutes up to 10 minutes
99407	Intensive, >10 minutes

These behavior change intervention codes are reported when the service is provided by a physician or other qualified health care professional. The service involves specific validated interventions, including assessing readiness for change and barriers to change, advising change in behavior, providing specific suggested actions and motivational counseling, and arranging for services and follow-up care. The medical record documentation must support the total time spent in performing the service, which may be reported in addition to other separate and distinct services on the same day.

The American Academy of Pediatrics publishes a complete line of coding publications, including an annual edition of *Coding for Pediatrics*. For more information on these excellent resources, visit the American Academy of Pediatrics Online Bookstore at **www.aap.org/bookstore/**.

Roadblocks
- Discuss and identify with the patient what they feel are the current barriers and help to identify solutions (eg, pharmacotherapies) that could address these roadblocks.

Repetition
- Discuss and use motivational techniques at every encounter. Encourage and remind patients that have failed attempts that most people make several attempts prior to cessation success, and that each time a cessation attempt is made, even if the attempt is unsuccessful, the tobacco user learns about cues to smoke, ways to combat the cues, and other lessons about quitting.

Another suggestion is to write a prescription for a 100% smoke- and tobacco-free home and car. This conveys a message to the family, including those members not at the medical visit, about the importance of creating completely smoke-free places. Changing the acceptability of smoking inside homes and cars can be an important step toward tobacco use cessation.

What Should You Do When You Identify Tobacco Smoke Exposure or Use?

- For patients and parents who use tobacco, follow the 5 As. Until the person quits, advise him or her to make their home and car smoke-free. Congratulate families for the efforts they are making to protect children from the harms of tobacco smoke exposure, and encourage them to continue to move toward quitting completely.

- For those who have quit, offer congratulations!

  - For those who quit during pregnancy, offer congratulations. Encourage them to stay quit after delivery, and offer support to help them stay quit.

- For those who are exposed to tobacco smoke, advise them to make their home smoke-free.

- For those who may be using tobacco periodically, advise them to stop before they become hooked.

What Results Should You Document?

Tobacco use and smoke exposure status of the family and household members should be documented, including former smoking status given the risk of relapse. Include in the problem list, summary list, and electronic medical record (EMR).

Follow up at every opportunity—develop a reminder system, either paper-based or EMR.

Resources

Aligne CA, Stoddard JJ. Tobacco and children: an economic evaluation of the medical effects of parental smoking. *Arch Pediatr Adolesc Med.* 1997;151(7):648–653

American Academy of Pediatrics Committee on Environmental Health, Committee on Substance Abuse, Committee on Adolescence, Committee on Native American Child Health. Policy statement—tobacco use: a pediatric disease. *Pediatrics.* 2009;124(5):1474–1487

Best D; American Academy of Pediatrics Committee on Environmental Health, Committee on Native American Child Health, Committee on Adolescence. Technical report—secondhand and prenatal tobacco smoke exposure. *Pediatrics.* 2009;124(5):e1017–e1044

Sims TH; American Academy of Pediatrics Committee on Substance Abuse. Technical report—tobacco as a substance of abuse. *Pediatrics.* 2009;124(5):e1045–e1053

Evidence-based Guidelines

Treating Tobacco Use and Dependence. Guideline products for consumers, primary care clinicians, specialists, health care administrators, insurers, and purchasers of insurance are available. See the Web site: http://www.surgeongeneral.gov/tobacco/. Also available at the Smoke Free Homes Program Web site.

Tools

Smoke Free Homes: The Professional's Toolbox: http://www.kidslivesmokefree.org/toolbox/

Books

US Department of Health and Human Services. *The Health Consequences of Involuntary Exposure to Tobacco Smoke: A Report of the Surgeon General.* Executive Summary. US Department of Health and Human Services, Centers for Disease Control and Prevention, Coordinating Center for Health Promotion, National Center for Chronic Disease Prevention and Health Promotion, Office on Smoking and Health; 2006

American Academy of Pediatrics Committee on Environmental Health. Environmental tobacco smoke and smoking cessation. In: Etzel RA, Balk SJ, eds. *Pediatric Environmental Health*. 2nd ed. Elk Grove Village, IL: American Academy of Pediatrics; 2003:147–163

Articles

27 Tobacco Use Health Indicators. Healthy People 2010. http://www.healthypeople.gov/default.htm

Web Sites

The AAP Richmond Center of Excellence: www.AAP.org/Richmondcenter
Provides materials and resources for pediatricians and other pediatric clinicians.

The Smoke Free Homes Program: http://www.kidslivesmokefree.org/
Provides materials and resources for pediatricians and other pediatric clinicians.

References

1. American Academy of Pediatrics Committee on Environmental Health, Committee on Substance Abuse, Committee on Adolescence, Committee on Native American Child Health. Tobacco use: a pediatric disease. *Pediatrics*. 2009;151(7):648–653

2. USDHHS. *The Health Consequences of Involuntary Exposure to Tobacco Smoke: A Report of the Surgeon General*. Atlanta, GA: US Department of Health and Human Services, Centers for Disease Control and Prevention, National Center for Chronic Disease Prevention and Health Promotion, Office on Smoking and Health; 2006

3. Fiore M, Jaen C, Baker T, et al. *Treating Tobacco Use and Dependence: 2008 Update. Clinical Practice Guideline*. Rockville, MD: US Department of Health and Human Services, Public Health Service; 2008

SANDRA G. HASSINK, MD
MARY LOU PULCINO, NP

WEIGHT MAINTENANCE AND WEIGHT LOSS

Bright Futures identifies healthy weight promotion as 1 of 2 critical themes within the guidelines. Recommendations in Bright Futures are consistent with the Prevention and Prevention Plus stages outlined in the Expert Committee Recommendations Regarding the Prevention, Assessment, and Treatment of Child Adolescent Overweight and Obesity.[1] With the widespread acceptance and dissemination of the Expert Committee Recommendations, coupled with the special significance Bright Futures places on healthy weight promotion, additional interventions included in the Expert Committee Recommendations are discussed.

Why Is It Important to Include Weight Maintenance and Weight Loss in Anticipatory Guidance?

Focusing on childhood obesity is now an urgent priority for pediatricians.[2] Almost one-third of children (31.7%) older than 2 years have a body mass index (BMI) greater than 85%,[3] 16.9% have a BMI greater than 95%, and 11.9% have a BMI greater than 97%. Almost 10% of children aged birth to 2 years have weight for height greater than the 95th percentile. There are differences in prevalence of overweight and obesity by age, with significant increases in BMI over the 85th, 95th, and 97th percentiles from toddlers to 6- to 11-year-olds. There was no significant difference in BMI percentiles between 6- to 11-year-olds and adolescents (Figure 1).[3]

While there is no difference between prevalence of obesity in boys and girls in the total population, Mexican-American boys were more likely to have higher BMIs at each BMI classification than Mexican-American girls, and Hispanic boys were more likely to have a BMI greater than 95% than Hispanic girls. There were no differences between non-Hispanic white and non-Hispanic black boys and girls.[3]

Figure 1.

BMI percentiles by age and gender

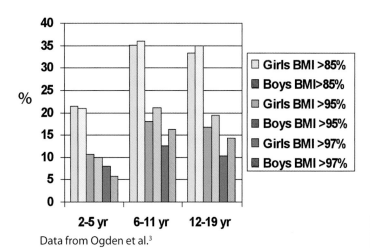

Data from Ogden et al.[3]

There are differences in prevalence of high BMI percentile by race/ethnicity. Hispanic boys were more likely to have a higher BMI than non-Hispanic white boys, and non-Hispanic black girls were more likely to have high BMIs than non-Hispanic white girls (Figure 2).[3]

There are persistent disparities "associated with socioeconomic status, school outcomes, neighborhoods, type of health insurance, and quality of care"[4] that will continue to need to be addressed.

ANTICIPATORY GUIDANCE

Figure 2.

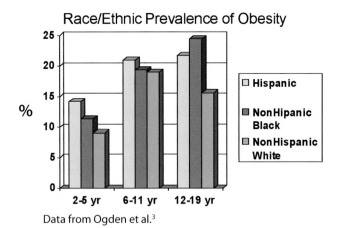

Race/Ethnic Prevalence of Obesity

Data from Ogden et al.[3]

Prevention is crucial because obesity is progressive. If untreated, a 13-year-old adolescent with a BMI greater than 95% has a 64% chance of being an obese 35-year-old, and chances of being an obese adult increase with the age of the obese teen.[5] Even more worrisome is that an obese 5-year-old has a 30% probability of becoming an obese adult,[5] and higher weight gain in the first 5 months of life has been correlated with obesity at 4.5 years.[6]

With another generation of obese children entering adulthood, health care costs for obesity-related illness continues to escalate, accounting for 9.1% of total health care spending in 2008.[7] The economic costs of obesity add to the cost to the child, family, and society of the loss of a healthy childhood. Obesity alters the trajectory of healthy growth and development in the domains of physical and mental health, emotional well-being, and psychosocial functioning.[1]

A whole host of obesity-related comorbidities, such as type 2 diabetes, polycystic ovarian syndrome, non-alcoholic steatohepatitis, hypertension lipid disorders, upper airway obstructive sleep apnea syndrome, Blount's disease, and slipped capital femoral epiphysis, affect obese children. Weight maintenance and weight loss are necessary to help prevent progression of these conditions.[1]

Should You Screen/Assess for Overweight or Obesity?

Body mass index screening is recommended for all children[1] as a first step toward universal obesity prevention and treatment. This means that all children should have BMI calculated and classified at every well-child visit. Bright Futures recommends assessing BMI for all children beginning at age 2 and plotting weight for length for children younger than 2. Body mass index screening should be incorporated into the office workflow with help from the office team. An electronic calculator, BMI table,[8] or BMI wheel can be used to calculate BMI, and BMI charts[8] can be used to classify BMI percentile. Severity categories are based on BMI, which is calculated from height and weight (wt [kg] /ht [m²] or wt [lbs]/ht [in] ² x 703) and plotted on BMI growth charts to obtain BMI percentile referenced to age and gender based on population data. The report recommended the classification of BMI percentiles as

- Underweight: less than 5th percentile

- Normal weight: 5th to 84th percentile

- Overweight: 85th to 94th percentile

- Obese: 95th to 99th percentile

- Morbid (severe) obesity: greater than 99th percentile

Classification of BMI category is the first step toward further assessment and treatment.

How Should You Screen/Assess for Overweight and Obesity?

In discussing obesity prevention and treatment, the Expert Committee Recommendations suggested a staged approach, which applied both to BMI classification and the resources needed to carry out obesity prevention and treatment.[1]

- **Prevention** is universal for children with BMI between the 5th and 84th percentile and includes review of healthy lifestyle behaviors, and the normal family risk, review of systems, and physical examination that would take place in the primary care office at well visits and other opportune visits.

- **Prevention plus** targets children with BMI between the 85th and 94th percentile classified as overweight and includes review of healthy lifestyle behaviors, family risk, review of systems, physical examination, and laboratory screening. Recommended labs include lipid panel with addition of fasting glucose and liver function studies if the child has additional risk factors. Practitioners should target any problem dietary and activity behaviors, review risks, and use patient-directed behavioral techniques to encourage lifestyle change. This intervention would occur in primary care practice and include monthly revisits.

- **Structured weight management** includes overweight children with health risk factors and children whose BMI is greater than 95% classified as obese.

  Evaluation includes review of healthy lifestyle behaviors, family risk, review of systems, physical examination, and laboratory screening. Recommended labs include lipid panel, fasting glucose and liver function studies, and other studies as clinically indicated. The practitioner would provide increased structure and goal setting, and could include referral to a dietitian or exercise specialist. This intervention could be a structured program or a series of structured revisits at the primary care level.

- **Comprehensive multidisciplinary interventions** would occur in a multidisciplinary obesity program, which could include a pediatrician, dietitian, exercise specialist, social worker, and mental health provider experienced in pediatric obesity. This stage would be for children who did not have success in previous stages and for children with severe obesity and/or obesity-related comorbidities, and would occur at a hospital clinic level.

- **Tertiary care intervention** occurs in the hospital setting for children with severe obesity and/or obesity-related comorbidities and includes a multidisciplinary obesity team as well as pediatric subspecialists. This intervention would be prepared to offer intense medical and surgical treatment and occur at the hospital level.

For all overweight/obese patients it is important to assess for obesity comorbidity risk in the family history and review of systems as well as signs and symptoms of obesity-related comorbidities. These findings can often provide motivation for families to change to healthier lifestyle behaviors. The American Academy of Pediatrics (AAP) *5-2-1-0 Pediatric Obesity Clinical Decision Support Chart* supports decision-making on assessment, evaluation, and laboratory testing.[8]

What Anticipatory Guidance Should You Provide if You Find Abnormal Results?

Prevention

All children in the BMI range from 5% to 84% should have prevention counseling at well visits and at any other opportune patient-physicians encounters. The content of this visit may be a review of the following:

- **5**—Consume at least 5 servings of fruits and vegetables daily.

- **2**—View no more than 2 hours of television per day. Remove televisions from children's bedrooms. No television viewing is recommended for children younger than 2.

- **1**—Be physically active at least 1 hour per day.

- **0**—Limit consumption of sugar-sweetened beverages (eg, soda and sports drinks).

It is also important to continue to encourage and promote maintenance of breastfeeding, which has a positive effect on obesity prevention[9] in addition to all its other benefits.

Beginning with the **5-2-1-0** message allows you to work with the family on considering what healthy lifestyle changes they are interested in trying, helping parents and children strategize about how to implement these changes, and working to set goals to measure progress.

Be positive and support small incremental steps for change.

Families find it helpful to have a reminder of their goals when they leave the visit (Figure 3).

Figure 3. Prescription for Healthy Active Living

R̲x̲ **for Healthy Active Living**

Name _____ Date _____

Ideas for Living a Healthy Active Life

5 Eat at least 5 fruits and vegetables every day.

2 Limit screen time (for example, TV, video games, computer) to 2 hours or less per day.

1 Get 1 hour or more of physical activity every day.

0 Drink fewer sugar-sweetened drinks. Try water and low-fat milk instead.

My Goals *(choose one you would like to work on first)*

☐ Eat _____ fruits and vegetables each day.

☐ Reduce screen time to _____ minutes per day.

☐ Get _____ minutes of physical activity each day.

☐ Reduce number of sugared drinks to _____ per day.

From Your Doctor

_____
Patient or Parent/Guardian signature

_____
Doctor signature

American Academy of Pediatrics
DEDICATED TO THE HEALTH OF ALL CHILDREN™

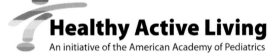
Healthy Active Living
An initiative of the American Academy of Pediatrics

Prevention plus is recommended for children with BMI between the 85th and 94th percentile for age and gender (overweight) and is structured to be provided in the primary care office setting. The most efficient way to provide this intervention is to use a team approach. For example, the person in the office who measures the height and weight may be the one to calculate and classify BMI, the office nurse may hand out a questionnaire to parents about healthy lifestyle behaviors, the physician may offer counseling and goal setting, and the check-out staff may ensure a timely revisit.

Behavior change begins with the provider helping the family/patient recognize the need for change by providing information about the child's current health status. It is important to assess willingness and capacity to change as a way of engaging the patient and family in moving toward action. Setting small achievable goals that work toward the desired behavior change helps patient and families succeed. Motivational interviewing is a technique that was recommended by the Expert Committee to help engage the family and patient in dialogue about change.[1]

The healthy eating and physical activity habits recommended for prevention plus in addition to **5-2-1-0** and breastfeeding include

- Prepare meals at home rather than eating at restaurants.

- Eat together as a family at the table at least 5 to 6 times per week.

- Eat a healthy breakfast daily.

- Include the entire family in making healthy lifestyle changes.

- Allow the child to self-regulate his/her meal when parents have provided a healthy meal in an appropriate portion size.

- Assist families in shaping recommendations to be consistent with their cultural values.

The goal for this stage is weight maintenance that with continued growth will reduce BMI. If after 3 to 6 months of monthly revisit the patient has not improved, proceed to Stage 2.

Structured Weight Management

The primary difference between prevention plus and structured weight management is that there is a specific plan to support the patient and family around behavior change. This could be carried out in a primary care office with additional support from a dietitian, counselor, physical therapist, or exercise therapist with training in pediatric obesity.

Goals for this stage include the goals as above for prevention plus in addition to

- ▶ Development of a plan for utilization of a balanced macronutrient diet emphasizing low amounts of energy-dense foods

- ▶ Increased structured daily meals and snacks

- ▶ Supervised active play of at least 60 per day

- ▶ Screen time of 1 hour or less per day

- ▶ Increased monitoring (eg, screen time, physical activity, dietary intake, restaurant logs) by provider, patient, and/or family

- This approach may be amenable to group visits with patient/parent component, nutrition, and structured activity.

- The goals for this stage are weight maintenance that decreases BMI as age and height increases. Weight loss should not exceed 1 lb/month in children aged 2 to 11 years, or an average of 2 lb/wk in older overweight/obese children and adolescents.

- If there is no improvement in BMI/weight after 3 to 6 months of monthly visits, the patient should be advanced to the next stage of comprehensive multidisciplinary intervention.

Comprehensive Multidisciplinary Intervention

This treatment usually is delivered in a pediatric weight management program by a multidisciplinary team composed of a behavioral counselor, a registered dietitian, an exercise specialist, and an obesity specialist.

Tertiary Care Intervention

This hospital-based intervention includes a multidisciplinary team providing care that includes a physician experienced in obesity management, a registered dietitian, behavioral counselor, and exercise specialist with expertise in childhood obesity and its comorbidities. Standard clinical protocols should be used for patient selection and evaluation before, during, and after intervention. Bariatric surgery, including gastric bypass or gastric banding, has shown to be effective but is available at only a few centers.

Obesity treatment can be successful.[10–14] Components of effective treatments have included dietary and physical activity interventions, behavioral therapy, family involvement, and access to multidisciplinary teams.[13,15] Key to building treatment capacity for pediatric obesity are reimbursement models that support multidisciplinary care, support for training the needed medical personnel, ongoing parenting and family support to sustain treatment effects, and continuing research into treatment effectiveness.

ICD9-CM Codes

The AAP obesity coding fact sheet[16] (available at aap.org/obesity) is a resource for practitioners and includes comprehensive coding information on obesity prevention and related comorbidities for practitioners.

Resources

Web Sites

Clinicians: American Academy of Pediatrics aap.org/obesity/health-professionals.html

Parents

HealthyChildren.org: http://www.healthychildren.org/English/health-issues/conditions/obesity/Pages/default.aspx

Families

American Academy of Pediatrics: http://www.aap.org/obesity/families_at_home.html

References

1. Barlow SE. Expert committee recommendations regarding the prevention assessment and treatment of child and adolescent overweight and obesity summary report. *Pediatrics.* 2007;120(suppl 4):S164–S192

2. Davis AMM, Gance-Cleveland B, Hassink S, Johnson R, Paradis G, Resnicow K. Recommendations for prevention childhood obesity. *Pediatrics.* 2007;120;S229–S253. http://www.pediatrics.org/cgi/content/full/120/Supplement_4/S164

3. Ogden CL, Carroll MD, Curtin LR, Lamb MM, Flegal KM. Prevalence of high body mass index in US children and adolescents, 2007–2008. *JAMA.* 2010;303(3):242–249

4. Bethell C, Simpson L, Stumbo S, Carle AC, Gombojav N. National, state, and local disparities in childhood obesity. *Health Aff (Millwood).* 2010;29(3):347–356

5. Guo SS, Wu W, Chumlea WC, Roche AF. Predicting overweight and obesity in adulthood from body mass index values in childhood and adolescence. *Am J Clin Nutr.* 2002;76:653–658

6. Dubois L, Girard M. Early determinants of overweight at 4.5 years in a population based longitudinal study. *Int J Obes.* 2006;30;610–617

7. Finkelstein EA, Trogdon JG, Cohen JW, Dietz W. Annual medical spending attributable to obesity; payer- and service-specific estimates. *Health Aff (Millwood).* 2009;28(5):w822–w831

8. American Academy of Pediatrics. Prevention and Treatment of Overweight and Obesity. American Academy of Pediatrics Web Site. http://www.aap.org/obesity/clinical_resources.html

9. Lamb MM, Dabelea D, Yin X, et al. Early life predictors of higher body mass index in healthy children. *Ann Nutr Metab.* 2010;56(1):16–22

10. Whitlock EA, O'Connor EP, Williams SB, Beil TL, Lutz KW. Effectiveness of weight management programs in children and adolescents. *Evid Rep Technol Assess (Full Rep).* 2008;(170):1–308

11. Nowicka P, Hoglund P, Pietrobelli A, Lissau I, Flodmark CE. Family weight school treatment; 1 year results in obese adolescents. *Int J Pediatr Obes.* 2008;3(3):141–147

12. Jelaltan E, Saelens IS. Empirically supported treatments in pediatric psychology; pediatric obesity. *J Pediatr Psychol.* 1999;24;223–248

13. American Dietetic Association. Position of the American Dietetic Association: individual-, family-, school-, and community-based interventions for pediatric overweight. *J Am Diet Assoc.* 2006;106:925–945

14. Garipagaoglu M, Sahip Y, Darendeliler F, Akdikemen O, Kopuz S, Sut N. Family-based group treatment versus individual treatment in the management of childhood obesity; randomized prospective clinical trail. *Eur J Pediatr.* 2009;168(9):1091–1099

15. US Preventive Services Task Force Screen for Obesity in Children and Adolescents. US Preventive Services Task Force recommendations statement. *Pediatrics.* 2010;125;361–367

16. American Academy of Pediatrics. Obesity and related co-morbidities coding fact sheet for primary care pediatricians. American Academy of Pediatrics Web site. http://www.aap.org/obesity/pdf/ObesityCodingFactSheet0208.pdf

INDEX

L

LAIV. *See* Live attenuated influenza vaccine (LAIV)
Late latent syphilis, 150
LDL cholesterol. See Low-density lipoprotein (LDL) cholesterol
Lead screening, 138–143
LEAP (Look to End Abuse Permanently), 30
Length/height, measuring, 52, 53–54
Lipids, 169
Lipid Screening and Cardiovascular Health in Children, 168, 172
Lipoproteins, 169
Literacy of parents, 39–43
Live attenuated influenza vaccine (LAIV), 145
Liver problems, 172
LoveisRespect.org, 31
Low-density lipoprotein (LDL) cholesterol, 169
Low-grade squamous intraepithelial lesion (LSIL), 115
LSIL. *See* Low-grade squamous intraepithelial lesion (LSIL)

M

M-CHAT. *See* Modified Checklist for Autism in Toddlers (M-CHAT)
Macrocephaly, 55
MAH. *See* Mental Health America (MAH)
MCV. *See* Meningococcal-conjugate vaccine (MCV)
Measles, mumps, rubella (MMR), 145
MedEdPPD.org, 37
Media usage, 163–165
Media violence, 163
Medial tibia stress syndrome, 94
Megalencephaly, 55
Meningitis, 142
Meningococcal-polysaccharide vaccine (MPSV), 145
Meningococcal-conjugate vaccine (MCV), 145
Menstrual irregularities, 172
Mental Health America (MAH), 23
Mental health screening, 18

Metabolic syndrome, 167. *See also* Cardiometabolic risk of obesity
Metatarsus varus, 77
Microcephaly, 55
Mixed hearing loss, 129, 135
MMR. *See* Measles, mumps, rubella (MMR)
Modified Checklist for Autism in Toddlers (M-CHAT), 125
Motivational interviewing, 175–177
MPSV. *See* Meningococcal-polysaccharide vaccine (MPSV)
Musculoskeletal history and examination, 94

N

NAFLD. *See* Nonalcoholic fatty liver disease (NAFLD)
NASH. *See* Nonalcoholic steatohepatitis (NASH)
National Center on Domestic and Sexual Violence, 31
National Coalition Against Domestic Violence (NCADV), 31
National Domestic Violence Hotline, 32
National Institute of Mental Health (NIMH), 23
National Teen Dating Abuse Helpline, 31–32
NCADV. *See* National Coalition Against Domestic Violence (NCADV)
Neurologic history and examination, 94
Newborn metabolic screening. *See* Immunizations, newborn screening, capillary blood tests
Newest Vital Sign (NVS), 40, 43
NICHQ-Vanderbilt ADHD Rating Scales, 22–23
Nicotine dependence, 45
Nicotine replacement options, 180
NIMH. *See* National Institute of Mental Health (NIMH)
Nonalcoholic fatty liver disease (NAFLD), 167
Nonalcoholic steatohepatitis (NASH), 172
NVS. *See* Newest Vital Sign (NVS)

O

OAE. *See* Otoacoustic emissions (OAE)
OARES, motivational interviewing components, 175–176
Obesity, 51, 57. *See also* Cardiometabolic risk of obesity; Weight maintenance/weight loss
Observation, 1. *See also* History, observation, and surveillance
Obstructive sleep apnea syndrome (OSAS), 172
ODD. See Oppositional defiant disorder (ODD)
Office for Victims of Crime (OVC), 32
Office on Violence Against Women (OVW), 31
OME. *See* Otitis media with effusion (OME)
Online PPD Support Group, 37
Opening the Mouth training program, 70
Oppositional defiant disorder (ODD), 17–23
Oral health, 65–73
Ortolani test, 89
OSAS. *See* Obstructive sleep apnea syndrome (OSAS)
Osgood-Schlatter disease, 94
Otitis media with effusion (OME), 130
Otoacoustic emissions (OAE), 131
Outtoeing, 75–77
OVC. *See* Office for Victims of Crime (OVC)
OVW. *See* Office on Violence Against Women (OVW)

P

PACT. *See* Protecting All Children's Teeth (PACT)
Pap test, 114
Parental health literacy, 39–43
Parents' Evaluations of Developmental Status (PEDS), 120, 122
Patella dislocation, 94
Patient Health Questionnaire-2 (PHQ-2), 37
Patient Health Questionnaire Adolescent Version (PHQ-A), 5, 7